Sparkling Praise for *Less Pain, Fewer Pills*

"Dr. Darnall has written a superb book for anyone suffering from chronic pain who needs alternatives to opiate medication. She has provided detailed cognitive-behavioral strategies that the patient can utilize to gain control over chronic pain. She also fully depicts the risks of chronic opiate therapy. The knowledge and skills she acquired in over 15 years of treating chronic pain patients are the cornerstones of this book."

—*John Loeser, MD*
Professor, University of Washington
Past President, American Pain Society and the
International Association for the Study of Pain

"Dr. Darnall offers a refreshing approach to sensible opioid-use reduction by considering the real issues facing patients today. I was particularly impressed that she did not set out to criticize opioids as a class, but rather articulated the conundrums and associated risks that prescribers and patients alike should understand before considering opioids acutely and chronically. More importantly she recognizes opioid usefulness balanced against important psychological vulnerabilities and non-medication strategies. She simplifies many of the issues without placing blame on patients with persistent pain or on clinicians. Overall, this book will help patients and providers understand the how and why of opioid prescription benefits versus risks. The importance of recognizing vulnerabilities and appropriately stratifying them is discussed; this will enable the patient-reader to take control of their prescribed medications and seek professional help if required, rather than falling victim to opioids controlling the outcome."

—*Jeffrey Fudin, BS, PharmD, FCCA*
Diplomate, American Academy of Pain Management
Owner & Managing Editor, PainDr.com & NovaPain Associates

"Every person with chronic pain can benefit from self-empowerment and the opportunity to reduce the need for drugs or medications. Dr. Darnall offers a critical review of chronic pain management and a thoughtful and pragmatic approach to self-empowerment — and to living with chronic pain in a manner that promotes as much personal wellbeing as is possible, ideally with fewer drugs and less pain."

—*Philip Pizzo, MD*
Former Dean and the David and Susan Heckerman Professor,
Stanford University School of Medicine

"Pain is a difficult symptom that is often over-treated by opioids, which in themselves lower the quality of life. This book gives great real-world examples and tips on how to avoid this vicious cycle. Beth Darnall is a leading expert in her field and has helped thousands of people with pain."

—*Kate Lorig, DrPH*
Director and Professor Emeritus, Patient Education Research
Center in the School of Medicine, Stanford University

"This book is a wonderful guide to help those suffering from chronic pain to not only understand the pitfalls of long-term opioid use, but more importantly to return to good health and everyday life activities. Dr. Beth Darnall's *Less Pain, Fewer Pills* offers readable and understandable advice to manage pain successfully while avoiding ineffective and harmful treatments, especially with opioids. For those suffering from unrelenting chronic pain, here is the guide that will make a difference."

—*Steven D. Feinberg, MD, MPH*
Board Certified, Physical Medicine & Rehabilitation
Board Certified, American Board of Pain Medicine
Past-President of the American Academy of Pain Medicine

"What we forget is that opioids don't simply dampen pain, they dampen everything—joy, energy, memory, social interactions, personality, life itself. If you want to fully experience life, you can—even if you have chronic pain — but not if you let opioids rule. Read this book and learn how to take back what you may have lost."

—*Jane C. Ballantyne, MD*
Professor of Education and Research; Director of the Pain Fellowship
University of Washington

"Dr. Darnall writes clearly and with empathy, and her balanced approach will help anyone struggling with chronic pain. This book provides patients with the tools they need to take back control of their pain and their lives without having to rely on pain medications."

—*Roger Chou, MD*
Associate Professor of Medicine, Oregon Health & Science University

"Dr. Darnall has created a book that eloquently articulates the perils of relying exclusively on opioids for the management of chronic pain. Through case studies and a very readable review of the scientific evidence, she makes a compelling case for utilizing non-opioids and behavioral therapies to manage ongoing pain. While this book is wholly accessible to lay readers, I would strongly encourage our medical colleagues, particularly those with substantial populations of pain patients to read this volume and to recommend it to their own patients and colleagues."

—*Robert Paul Cowan, MD, FAAN*
Professor of Neurology, Stanford University School of Medicine
Director, Stanford Headache Program

"Dr. Darnall's new book provides a refreshing approach to reduce reliance on prescription opioids for chronic pain. The book not only provides an accurate description of the problems related to long-term opioid use—it also presents an effective, step-by-step approach to eliminate the use of prescription opioids."

—*Michael W. Hooten, MD*
Division of Pain Medicine,
Mayo Clinic, Rochester, Minnesota

Less Pain
FEWER PILLS

Less Pain
FEWER PILLS

*Avoid the dangers of prescription opioids
and gain control over chronic pain*

Beth Darnall, PhD

Bull Publishing Company
Boulder, Colorado

Bull Publishing Company
P.O. Box 1377
Boulder, CO USA 80306
www.bullpub.com

Library of Congress Cataloging-in-Publication Data

Darnall, Beth.

Less pain, fewer pills : avoid the dangers of prescription opioids and gain
  control over chronic pain / Beth Darnall, PhD.

   pages cm

Summary: "For sufferers of chronic pain, the author provides the best
chronic pain treatment options that work over time and carry the least risk.
This book gives the information and tools needed to meet this challenge--
to take responsibility for and proactively manage your own pain on your
own terms for the rest of your life"-- Provided by publisher.

ISBN 978-1-936693-58-0 (paperback)

1. Chronic pain--Alternative medicine--Popular works. 2. Self-care,
Health--Popular works. I. Title.

RB127.D39 2014

616'.0472--dc23

                                                        2014013064

Printed in U.S.A.

22 21 20 19 18   10 9 8 7 6 5 4 3

Interior design and production by Dovetail Publishing Services
Cover design and production by Shannon Bodie, Lightbourne, Inc.

Contents

Preface

At least 100 million Americans—or about one-third of the population—suffer from chronic, often debilitating pain. It's a surprising statistic and it's directly related to the widespread overprescribing of drugs such as Vicodin, oxycodone, and other potentially harmful pain medications.

Prior to the 1990s, opioid medications* (Vicodin and oxycodone being the most well-known examples) were mostly used to treat short-term pain as a consequence of surgery, injury, or the pain caused by cancer. Typically, these pain relief medications were not recommended to treat chronic pain that extended beyond a 90-day period.

But in the early 1990s physicians began allowing their patients to continue using these medications for indefinite periods, often for years on end. While some people with chronic pain improved, on average, prescribing practices had jumped ahead of any good science showing that the long-term use of opioids was beneficial for most people with chronic pain. The long-term consequences to individual health—and by extension, society at large—remained largely unexplored. This book pulls back the veil on the individual and societal consequences of these approaches to pain management that often are ineffective at best, and at worst harmful to a patient's long-term health.

---

*Opioid medications are commonly referred to as "painkillers." I minimize use of this term because in the context of chronic pain it conveys a false message: that chronic pain can be "killed" or eradicated with a pill.

While simple medical problems such as a bacterial infection can be solved by prescribing medication that kills the bacteria, chronic pain is a complex problem that cannot be solved with such a simple pill-based medical approach. In fact, a solely pill-based approach can lead to more problems. Successful chronic pain treatment and management can often be achieved without opioids. And, if opioids are prescribed, successful chronic pain management requires a balanced approach that includes the use of opioids as just one part of a comprehensive, holistic pain care management plan. Yet in the past 10 years the number of opioid prescriptions has increased by 400 percent, making them the most widely prescribed class of drugs in the United States. In fact, in 2011 more than 238 million opioid prescriptions were filled in the United States alone.[1]

Readers of this book will learn how to use these medications mindfully to avoid the hidden health pitfalls that accompany opioids—even when they are taken exactly as prescribed. It is well known that opioids are subject to addiction and abuse by those seeking an opioid "high"—a subject which many books address. But this book focuses on other hidden health risks that are relevant to everyone who takes prescription opioids for pain.

In the past few decades there has been a steep trend of prescribing opioids to treat chronic pain with little understanding of the health risks. If you (or your doctor) do not know about the risks associated with opioids, you may be set up for problems down the road. And if you do not use nonopioid pain management strategies, you may be unwittingly overrelying on opioids and exposing yourself to opioid risks to a greater degree. Armed with the right information, you can make informed decisions about your pain care. You can learn to reduce your own pain and suffering, thereby improving your health and well-being.

As a pain psychologist who has treated chronic pain exclusively for almost 15 years, I have helped countless motivated patients find their own path to either leaving opioid use behind or at least reducing use so that these medications are just one component of a comprehensive, individual pain care management plan.

If you have chronic pain, this book and the tools I provide will guide you toward building your treatment plan so that you rely less or not at all on opioids to manage your pain. The skills you learn and use will give you greater control over your physical, mental, and emotional experience.

At the same time, I hope the information in this book will allow you to add a moderating voice to calls from both public and private groups who wish to greatly restrict access to all opioids. Yes, there are real risks to patients who choose to use these medications, but it is woefully shortsighted to take away opioids without giving those in pain other ways to help themselves. Patients must be given the opportunity to discover better ways to care for themselves so that, ultimately, they don't need opioids, or at least they use less of them. As a pain management professional, I believe that the best chronic pain treatment options are the ones that work over time and carry the least risk. If you suffer from chronic pain, I hope this book gives you the information and tools you need to meet this challenge—and proactively manage your own pain on your own terms for the rest of your life.

Acknowledgments

My sincere gratitude goes to Melanie Thernstrom, PhD, my gifted editor, whose expertise and advisement absolutely transformed this project. Melanie is the *New York Times* bestselling author of *The Pain Chronicles*, and she lent expertise and counsel that extended well beyond her title as editor on this project.

I also want to extend my appreciation to Jim Bull for believing in the topic and in me, and to Claire Cameron and Emily Sewell at Bull Publishing for their incredible skill and support.

My heartfelt thanks and appreciation to the following people, who also had a direct impact on the development, completion, and publication of this book: Sean Mackey, MD, PhD; Ken Flummer; Kate Lorig, PhD; Don Freeman; Nita Bryant; Steven Forrest; Meredith Barad, MD; Mark Wallace, MD; Scott Fishman, MD; Sheena Aurora, MD; Michael Leong, MD; Brett Stacey, MD; Julio Gonzalez, MD; Michael Schatman, PhD; Joe DeAngelis; Keith Boettiger; Ming-Chih Kao, PhD, MD; Jeffrey Anderson, MD; Mark Morrow; and Dovetail Publishing Services.

Finally, I dedicate the book to the countless clients I have worked with, whose stories and courage inspired me to write so that others might suffer less.

Instead of national initiatives that focus on opioid legislation and opioid dose limitations, I dream of a national health care initiative aimed at giving the people with chronic pain the tools to control their pain experience, their health, and their lives.

PART I
The Problem

One Girl's Story

The girl had wrenching stomach pain for as long as she could remember. It was a pain that would come and go without rhyme or reason and lord over her life like an uninvited narcissistic relative showing up at her door. When the pain visited her it demanded her attention.

Although the girl had spent her life dealing with these unwanted pain visitations, she knew very little about their source but was well aware of the direct impact on her life. Eating and even breathing were difficult when the pain arrived. All she could do in response to these bouts of pain was to lie in a quiet room and wait for the razor-sharp stabs in her stomach to subside to a more tolerable level that felt something like churning needles of pain.

What was so perplexing to the girl was that these random pain attacks stood in stark contrast to the rest of her life. She was a competitive athlete, she was socially engaged with her peers, and she had a work ethic some might describe as obsessive. All through her childhood she was never evaluated for this pain or its root causes. Instead, she dealt with the pain silently and alone. Then a tragic event happened when she was 18. The death of her boyfriend pushed her to the edge of her coping skills. She was away at college, a thousand miles from home.

"Mom, my stomach is killing me," she told her mother over the phone, her voice full of desperation and fear as she recounted her symptoms. "It's never been this bad. It hurts to breathe. What if it gets worse?" Uncharacteristically, she burst into tears. Her mother, who could do nothing directly for her, urged her to get help. With a long-standing line of stoicism now finally breached, she called for a taxi and frantically told the driver to take her to the nearest emergency room.

She wasn't sure exactly what to expect when she walked into the emergency room of her university's hospital, but she desperately hoped the doctors would finally be able to explain her pain and offer her a cure that would fix the problem once and for all.

All of the standard tests—blood screens, X-rays, and physical examinations—came back negative. While the doctors offered her no answers about the cause of the pain, they gave her one thing: a prescription for Vicodin. So the girl went home and took the medication--exactly as she was prescribed to do.

The year was 1990. The girl who was rushed to the hospital in a taxi was me.

❧   ❦

I never received treatment for the underlying issues that had caused my pain—likely a combination of food sensitivities, a reaction to traumatic experience, and chronic stress, with a bit of undiagnosed irritable bowel disorder on the side. And within this soup of possible causes and diagnosis is the point.

Clearly, I had some medical problem that was being aggravated by my body's reaction to the stress I was creating by worrying about the pain and its source (i.e., catastrophizing it). In other words, rather than coping with the pain, I was reacting to the pain, and this reaction was one of a combination of factors that joined forces to create my pain cycles. Had I not learned other ways to resolve my bouts with pain I might still be taking opioids today, even though studies show that opioids are not an effective treatment option for the sources of my pain.

After leaving the emergency room that day, I continued taking Vicodin for about 8 months, and I did find relief in the soothing numbness it brought to my life. In many ways, the medication provided a welcome vacation from mourning the loss of someone I loved and struggling to keep my focus on class assignments. Eventually, I began to take the pills before I really needed them to "stay ahead of the pain." At the time this seemed a perfectly reasonable decision since my primary care physician at the student health clinic kept writing prescriptions.

Over time—and on my own—I arrived at the conclusion that Vicodin was not helping me. I noticed my choices and my reactions were different when I was taking opioids. I felt spacey and passive and eventually concluded that I just wasn't quite myself anymore. So, without talking to my doctor or anyone else, I stopped taking the medication and self-prescribed a new treatment.

The new plan forced me to finally deal with the factors that led to my pain becoming unmanageable in the first place. This difficult process truly changed my life. It deepened my self-awareness and prepared me for a future of helping others caught in this cycle of medication-centered pain management.

Eventually, I became a specialist in chronic pain psychology whose practice approaches pain management in a holistic way by focusing not just on the physical symptoms but also on the person dealing with the pain. This approach means that I give my patients full information about the risks and benefits of taking opioid medications and encourage them to make informed decisions about using these medications. And if a patient decides to seek pain relief using opioids, I provide guidance on how to need as little of the medication as possible. It's an approach that I recommend no matter what type of pill is involved. For me the simple fact is this: taking fewer pills should always be the goal.

Clearly, minimizing the number of pills or avoiding them altogether to manage pain differently is one of the main goals of this book. *Less Pain* is designed to put its reader in charge, just as I put my patients in charge. Part I of the book (chapters 1–4) presents the problems associated with the exclusive use of opioids to control pain and shows readers how to make an informed choice about using medications. Part II (chapters 5–11) focuses on what you can do to reduce your pain to avoid or reduce the need for pain medication. These techniques include ways to calm your nervous system and reduce your suffering, as well as different ways of thinking about pain. You'll also learn about choices you can make that support reclaiming control of your life. With this information as background, this book will show you how to develop a personalized pain control program—your empowerment program.

I wrote this book to share the techniques that helped transform my life and the lives of the many clients* I work with every day in my clinic. I am convinced, based on my experience and those of my clients, that the techniques in this book will change your life as well.

---

*Throughout the book I use the terms 'patient' and 'client' interchangeably. Like most psychologists, I prefer the term client because it is empowering and minimizes a focus on sickness. However, multidisciplinary medical settings involve team conferences and discussions about 'patient care' and the term 'patient' is interwoven into daily parlance. For this reason many pain psychologists may use the term 'patient' rather than client.

A Painkiller Trap?

IN 2013 THE CENTERS FOR DISEASE CONTROL reported that the amount of opioid prescriptions sold in 2010 was enough to medicate every US adult with a typical dose of 5 mg of hydrocodone every 4 hours for 1 month. These startling figures represent a 300 percent increase in the sales rate over 11 years.[2]

What is going on? Why the striking increase in opioid prescriptions? Has the opioid prescription boom helped people with chronic pain? Are patients actually getting better? What are the medical risks that come with long-term opioids? What are the psychological risks? Do patients understand these risks? Can we reduce opioid prescriptions by treating chronic pain better? These are the questions I set out to investigate.

People take opioids because they want their pain to be better managed and they may mistakenly believe opioids will make their pain go away. In fact, when it comes to chronic pain, opioids offer limited pain relief. Without knowing about the limitations of opioids, people may fall into the trap of taking *more* opioids in an effort to achieve a mythical "pain-free" life.

If you take opioids, you have not done something wrong nor have you failed. Indeed, it is possible to take these medications mindfully as *one part* of your pain care plan. And once you learn the skills that empower you to need and use less medication, you'll be one step closer to the goal of shrinking your pain without pills and avoiding some of the serious medical problems associated with opioids.

Why Are Opioids Overprescribed?

Physicians, nurses, and other prescribers* often struggle to manage the complexities of patients who have chronic pain. The average prescriber of opioids is a generalist—often a primary care physician—and not a pain specialist. Many general physicians have a limited understanding of the full range of opioid risks, and they may be unaware of the alternatives. You might reasonably expect your doctor to tell you if there is something different or better than opioids, but many doctors don't know this information because chronic pain is not covered well in medical school, if at all.

A 2011 study found pain education is "fragmented," delivered to medical students in bits and pieces in the midst of courses that focus on specific diseases, such as arthritis or cancer, rather than as a stand-alone topic. As recently as 2011, fewer than 4 percent of medical schools reported having a required pain course, and these pain courses ranged from 1.5 to 13 days. Less than one in five US medical schools even offered a pain elective. Many US medical schools did not teach any dedicated pain courses, and many others committed fewer than 5 *hours* to pain education over 4 years. Now consider that your

---

*In addition to medical doctors (MDs), registered nurses (RNs) and advanced practice registered nurses (APRNs) can prescribe medications independently, but state law determines whether opioids may be prescribed. Physician assistants (PAs) can prescribe under the license of an MD, but certain states do not allow them to prescribe opioids. Many types of nurse specialists have prescribing privileges that vary by license and state.

physician or prescriber probably completed medical school well before this study took place, when pain education was further lacking. Moreover, the psychology of pain—a critical aspect of chronic pain that influences pain and the prescription and use of opioids—is not taught at all.[3,4]

Poor medical education for pain extends to Europe, too. A recent survey of European primary care doctors* found that 90 percent were dissatisfied with their initial training in chronic pain treatment. Up to 46 percent reported discomfort in prescribing opioids for chronic pain due to lack of training.[5]

While pain is the most common reason people visit their family doctor, care providers have been placed in the unfair situation of treating people with chronic pain when they are inadequately trained to do so. Doctor surveys suggest that after completing primary care residency training, half of doctors feel only "somewhat prepared" to counsel their patients about pain. Close to one-third of doctors surveyed reported feeling "somewhat unprepared" or "very unprepared." It is no wonder that physicians, nurse practitioners, and physician assistants report discomfort in treating chronic pain.*

For doctors treating chronic pain, opioid education focuses on the specifics of prescribing, policing, and monitoring medication use. Often the emphasis is on catching addiction or on protecting the doctor from legal repercussions—all while omitting the most important information: what can a patient do to better manage their pain *themselves,* without a pill?

With many primary care doctor visits lasting 15 minutes or less—sometimes much less—it's easy to see why the appointment is focused on writing a prescription. Often, what gets left out are the discussions about lasting alternatives to prescriptions and critical education about any medications being prescribed. The following

---

*From this point forward I will consolidate all prescribers (RN, PA, MD, etc.) into the terms doctor or physician for ease of language and readability.

story illustrates just some of the problems that can arise when the focus remains on pills alone.

☙ ❧

Jaqui's Story

One day I received a call from a primary care physician I know very well, Dr. Bower. "Beth, I have a patient I am hoping you can see. She has chronic back and neck pain that's been worsening; she's on opioids and seems to be unraveling. She's asking me to increase her dose again, and I'm not comfortable with that. Is there any chance you can see her in the next few weeks?"

Within the week Jaqui was sitting in my office. She was 36, married, and had two sons, ages 4 and 2. She took a short-term medical leave when she began having trouble keeping up with the duties of her administrative assistant job due to back and neck pain. Overwhelmed, she called Dr. Bower—the person who was supposed to fix her pain. When Dr. Bower denied her request for more hydrocodone, Jaqui went into an emotional tailspin. "What am I going to do?" she thought. "I won't be able to work." Then she began having panic attacks.

Almost as soon as she sat in my office she began crying. "All I wanted was help with my pain," she said as she wiped her face with a tissue. "Now Dr. Bower either thinks I'm a head case or she thinks I'm a drug seeker. I'm not sure which."

I assured Jaqui that neither was the case. Dr. Bower just wanted to find the best treatment pathway for her, and it wasn't clear that more opioids would help. Jaqui didn't see it that way. "My pain is *worse* and I can't work," she said. "I don't understand how more medication wouldn't help that."

I nodded. "Let's take a step back so I can learn more about you, your history, and what's going on now," I said.

I learned that Jaqui's back and neck pain began 2 years ago following a car accident. At the time, she was 7 months pregnant with her youngest son, Caleb. Her 2-year-old son, Nathan, was in the car with her when the crash happened. Nathan was fine—he had been riding in his car seat. Terrified about the health of her baby, Jaqui rushed to the hospital. She had trouble breathing on the way there and felt shaky as her heart raced. She was told these were signs that she was having a panic attack. Jaqui was relieved to learn that her baby was healthy. She was told she had whiplash and was prescribed opioids.

Most whiplash pain resolves in a few weeks, but Jaqui's pain never really improved. She had trouble sleeping. She found herself worrying about things—mostly about the safety of her children—so she tossed and turned for hours before falling asleep. Her pain would also wake her up during the night. The physical demands of a baby put further strain on her neck and back.

Her pain became chronic, and Dr. Dower refilled her opioid prescriptions every month. She took one OxyContin in the morning to help her get going, another in the afternoon when her pain seemed to get worse. Recently, at bedtime she began taking more opioids that were prescribed to her "as needed for pain." She also found the opioids helped calm her mind so she could settle into sleep. Right away I understood that, in part, Jaqui was taking opioids to help her anxiety.

To her credit, Jaqui had met her goal of returning to work 8 months earlier, but the transition was fraught with difficulties, more pain, and a request for more medication. Jaqui chalked up her pain to the workday: she was commuting, sitting all day, and unable to take care of herself like she did when she was home with the kids. But I suspected there might be more to the story.

"How did you feel when you went to work and left your boys at day care?"

She winced. "Terrible. My husband, Tom, would take them to day care, and I would have him call me once they were safely out of the car." Even though her boys were not injured in the car accident, Jaqui had been imprinted with fear for their safety—especially when it came to driving. She didn't think about it too much during the day, but at night when she went to bed and had no other distractions, fears about her boys would creep into her mind and sometimes stay for an hour or more.

Despite her pain and anxiety, Jaqui held it together until 2 weeks ago when she called Dr. Bower for more medication because her pain was worse again. I asked her if anything stressful had happened. She took a deep breath. "I had a near-miss while driving with the boys." A car suddenly darted into her lane. Perhaps it wasn't that close of a call—she couldn't be sure—but she slammed hard on the brakes and everyone was scared. The boys began crying and then so did she. She realized that in her own hasty reaction she could have killed them all.

Nobody was hurt and the boys quickly calmed down. Jaqui, on the other hand, was badly shaken up. The incident stoked her fears, muscle tension, and pain. She could no longer manage at work. She began worrying that she might have reinjured her neck.

When Dr. Bower denied her request for more opioids, Jaqui was bewildered. "What am I supposed to do? Suffer? I need to work! All I have ever been given for pain is opioids and now suddenly it's wrong?"

Whether opioids were right or wrong for Jaqui is debatable, but it was clear that opioid medication alone was not helping her. I could see, in fact, it was causing her problems. Her increasing anxiety was worsening her pain—and her distress about her pain—and it was leading to opioid dose escalation. The overfocus on the opioids was actually compounding her anxiety because the only thing that reduced her distress was a pill. Now she was fretting about her boys, her pain, *and* making sure she had prescriptions and enough pain medication!

Jaqui needed comprehensive pain care that, at minimum, included a pain psychologist, a physical therapist, and a pain physician. These appointments were made while I worked with Jaqui to address her underlying anxiety. The anxiety was increasing her distress about her pain, and it was preventing her from getting the rest that helps keep pain low. Reducing her anxiety about driving helped her to relax and be more focused behind the wheel so she was less likely to overreact. As she became calmer, her muscle tension began to melt away and her pain lessened. In physical therapy she learned exercises to build strength in certain muscles, and this helped her pain and flexibility. She was cleared for a daily exercise program, and she was surprised that regular exercise—something she had avoided out of fear it would worsen her pain—actually eased it! Exercise also helped her anxiety and her sleep. Her pain physician prescribed a nonopioid pain medication—duloxetine—that was better suited for her specific type of pain. We started Jaqui on an opioid taper, and in a few months she was off opioids completely.

Everybody was happy. Jaqui was thrilled because her life was better. She was no longer desperate to find relief in a pill bottle, and she no longer felt like a hostage to her doctor and the prescriptions. Dr. Bower was equally pleased because her patient was getting the right treatment, their healthy doctor-patient relationship had been restored, and Jaqui's health was now steadily improving. It was also exciting for me to watch Jaqui gain control over her pain and her life through the use of the empowering techniques she learned in our sessions.

❦

The standard medical practice of writing a prescription for a medical problem and sending a patient on their way does not work well with chronic pain. Prescriptions alone do not address the complexities of chronic pain.

Chronic pain is a complex problem. There are usually many reasons why a person's pain starts and many factors that shape and maintain the pain. And although medications may help to lessen pain, such therapies rarely cure chronic pain.

In my work, I focus on improving quality of life, which requires treating the whole person and not just their pain. Research shows that the outcomes for patients taking long-term opioids for chronic pain are poor unless paired with other treatments, such as the ones discussed in this book.

We would like to think that pain care in the United States is of the highest quality. The United States, which constitutes less than 5 percent of the world's population, consumes 80 percent of the entire world production of opioids and 99 percent of the global supply of hydrocodone.* However, opioids alone are not a cure-all treatment for chronic pain. Every country has challenges in treating pain, but the United States is perhaps unique in that chronic pain is often overtreated with opioids and undertreated in other ways that are generally more effective. We need to treat the underlying factors that make pain worse and lead to increased need for opioids and other medications.

At What Cost Are Opioids Overprescribed?

The surge in opioid prescribing has propelled opioids to become the most widely prescribed class of drugs in the United States. In 2011, hydrocodone, known by the brand name Vicodin, held the dubious distinction of being the single most commonly prescribed medication in the United States, with 137 million prescriptions written.*

More than 10 million Americans take opioids at least once a week. More than 4 million Americans take opioids regularly, defined as 5 days a week for at least 4 weeks.† Among regular opioid users, almost half have been taking opioids for 2 years or longer, and nearly one-fifth have been taking opioids for 5 years or more.

US prescribers are more inclined to treat chronic pain with opioids than *any other place in the world*, including Europe, where opioids have generally been reserved for cancer pain. However, some of the grave problems seen in the United States may emerge in other countries as opioid prescribing gains traction. For instance, Germany had a 37 percent increase in opioid prescriptions between 2000 and

---

*Sloan Epidemiology Center.

†Manchikanti, L., Fellows, B., Ailinani, H, Pampati, V. Therapeutic use, abuse and nonmedical use of opioids: a ten-year perspective. *Pain Physician 2010*. 13(5):401-35.

2010, with more than three-quarters of those prescriptions written for chronic pain. Of particular concern is the increase in prescribing potent, immediate-release opioids for chronic pain, given the general lack of benefit.[6] The overemphasis on opioids means that other strategies are often minimized—strategies that may work better in the long run, have fewer risks, and allow people to use less medication overall. As more prescriptions are written, more people are being exposed to the risks that come with taking their opioids exactly as prescribed. And more opioids are finding their way to the streets and being sold and used illegally with tragic and even fatal consequences.

How Did Opioid Prescriptions Become an Epidemic?

Before the 1990s, opioid prescribing in the United States was similar to European prescribing practices. Opioids were prescribed almost exclusively for the short period of time needed to bridge a patient's comfort level while they healed from a major injury, surgery, or dental procedure. Then things started to change. Doctors began expanding use of opioids to treat chronic pain—pain that might have no end in sight.

Unfortunately, physicians did not have good information about the risks associated with the long-term use of these medications. The misinformation was the result of an aggressive marketing campaign by the pharmaceutical industry that targeted patients and physicians, and exaggerated the benefits of opioids while downplaying the risks. Physicians began writing more opioid prescriptions because they believed that they were properly treating their patients' chronic pain. They based their belief on the message they were hearing:

What's good for *short*-term pain is also good for *long*-term pain. The truth: Opioids are good treatment for a minority of people with chronic pain—a small subset of people who become more active, more functional, and have better quality of life with few negative side effects over the long run.

Unfortunately, no early studies were conducted to determine exactly who is best suited for opioid therapy and who is most at risk for the negative effects of opioids. The very few existing studies were conducted over 2–6 *weeks*—too short a time for many of the risks to manifest. As a result, the short-term studies declared opioids to be safe and effective for long-term use when in fact there had been no long-term studies. People who take opioids for chronic pain often take them for years or even decades, which leads to entirely different risks than short-term use.

The long-term studies conducted since that time show that opioids are a questionable treatment for chronic pain.[7] And while a common perception remains that opioids provide strong pain relief, the few trials that compared opioids to nonsteroidal anti-inflammatory drugs (NSAIDs) or antidepressants found that opioids provided the same level of relief for chronic back pain.[8] However, all these studies share the problem of being less than 6 months in length[7]—far shorter than the average length of time opioids are prescribed for chronic pain.

The value of the early opioid studies was further limited by the fact that they excluded anyone who suffered from anxiety or depression, or who was not taking many other medications. In real life almost everyone who has chronic pain either has depression or anxiety, or is taking multiple medications, so the results from the early studies cannot be generalized to the average patient. Simply put, the early studies did not provide doctors with the information they needed to make good treatment decisions for people who have chronic pain.

The pharmaceutical industry actively targeted primary care physicians to encourage them to prescribe opioids for chronic pain by advertising half-truths in medical journals and by publishing data that falsely declared opioids carry less than a 3 percent risk for addiction.* Although some physicians were paid spokespersons and others

---

*The appendix provides a broader historical synopsis of the pharmaceutical industry's role in opioid overprescribing in the United States, as documented in the 2003 report from the US Governmental Accounting Office.

received incentives such as lunches and other perks from the pharmaceutical companies, many physicians prescribed opioids because they truly believed it was the best care for chronic pain. The majority of physicians trusted what they were being told.

The FDA has recognized that, in part, doctors have overprescribed opioids because they had very little information about the real risks for long-term use in chronic pain. In response to the so-called epidemic, in 2013 the US Food and Drug Administration stated that it would require drug companies to conduct longer-term studies on extended-release and long-acting opioids.

The tendency to overprescribe opioids was also fueled by the fact that physicians were under increasing pressure to eliminate pain. In 2001 a campaign was waged by the Joint Commission* to include pain as the "fifth vital sign" in patient care. The four vital signs measured at each medical visit include heart rate, blood pressure, body temperature, and respiratory rate. As the fifth vital sign, at *every* medical visit patients were now being asked to rate their pain level.† Education efforts informed patients that they had a right to adequate pain control, which many patients interpreted as a right to be pain-free. Suddenly there was a flood of people needing—indeed, demanding—pain treatment from doctors who had limited pain education and few treatment options, and felt an obligation to "fix" their patient's pain.'

---

*The Joint Commission is an independent, not-for-profit organization that accredits and certifies health care organizations in the United States.

†In adults, pain is typically measured by asking patients to rate how intense their pain is on a 0–10 scale (where 0 = no pain and 10 = worst pain imaginable) or on a 0–100 scale (where 0 = no pain and 100 = worst pain imaginable). For children or adults with limited cognitive ability, clinicians use the Wong-Baker faces pain scale, which is composed of six faces that depict progressive expressions of discomfort and distress. Patients are asked to point to the face that best describes how they are feeling at that moment. For nonverbal individuals, clinicians observe pain behaviors and use blood pressure and pulse as indices of current pain.

Why Don't Opioids Work for Many People with Chronic Pain?

Many people believe that taking an opioid "painkiller" will make them pain-free. After all, it eliminated their pain after in their surgery, dental procedure, or injury. And opioids do lift pain in the beginning—just long enough for patients to pin their hopes on them. But they don't cure pain: research shows that even when taking opioids for up to 8 weeks, on average opioids reduce pain by about 25–30 percent[9]—a far cry from pain-free. And bear in mind that these studies were conducted during the early "honeymoon" weeks when opioids are working best. Over the ensuing months so-called **tolerance*** develops: opioid medication becomes less effective, and higher doses are needed to achieve the same amount of pain relief. And those higher doses naturally increase the negative side effects of opioids.

If you take prescription opioids long term, you are likely to experience negative side effects, regardless of whether they improve your pain.

In fact, 80 percent of people with chronic pain who take opioids report negative side effects and unexpected problems from using opioid medication *exactly as prescribed*.[9,10] Once you learn about your specific risks, you will be motivated to use as little opioid medication as possible—or you may decide that it is simply not worth it.

Some of the side effects of opioids are noticeable and may show up early on. These are easier to catch and easier to link to the medications. However, other side effects are not easily detected because they evolve slowly. As a result, it's harder to make the connection between the new

---

*This and many other terms in bold type appear in the glossary.

problem and the opioid. This may lead doctors and patients to inflate the "benefit" of the opioids because the true risk or "cost" goes unnoticed.

Opioid medication can change your brain and the chemistry of your body in a way that can lead to more pain and more problems. Among other things, opioids cause imbalances in your body when used long term. Opioids lower hormone levels such as testosterone and estrogen, and this can lead to mood problems, sleep problems, and even increased pain. Opioids prevent you from reaching some of the deeper stages of sleep, and this can leave you feeling more fatigued and in greater pain the following day. These disturbances and imbalances create *new* problems, which are often treated with *more* medications. The result: an increasingly complex medical picture that places patients at risk for more side effects caused by the new pills (see Figure 2.1).

Most people taking prescription opioids were not adequately warned of the risks at the outset. In the past, good research did not exist, and doctors and patients alike remained in the dark about the risks, even as opioid prescriptions climbed. But more is known now, and the evidence is disturbing. Increasingly, patients with chronic pain, angry at how their health status has worsened or been

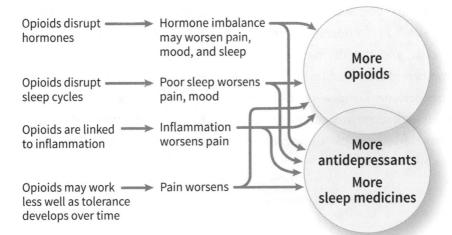

Figure 2.1   How opioids can lead to more pain and more medications

complicated by opioids, say to me, "Nobody told me about these risks and problems." I empathize: People have every right to be angry.

It is important for you and your doctor to carefully consider *your specific risks* before you begin taking prescription opioids.

Opioids affect individuals differently. Your opioid risks depend on whether you are male or female, how old you are, your pain condition, your other medical problems, other medications you are taking, whether you are depressed or anxious or have any other mental health problems, and whether or not you have a history of substance abuse. For example, a depressed 22-year-old woman who once struggled with alcohol abuse will have opioid risks that are entirely different from those of a 77-year-old man with a heart condition. In fact, opioid risks vary so widely between individual patients that it is as if each patient is taking a completely different medication.

It is critical that you and your doctor understand *your specific risks*—only then can you calculate whether your opioid risks outweigh any possible benefits. In order to make an informed choice, you must first understand not only your risks but the limitations of opioids, and the alternatives.[11,12] I find that once patients understand that opioids may reduce their pain by only about 25 percent—and over time perhaps far less—*and* once they consider their health risks, they often seek alternative strategies that can be more effective with lasting results. Most people are eager to find ways to gain independence from the pill bottle.

Know Your Specific Risks

Knowledge Is Power: Protect Yourself and Minimize Your Risk

THERE IS CONTROVERSY ABOUT the use of opioids for chronic pain, particularly given the associated risks, both known and unknown.[13,14] While many medicines used to treat chronic conditions have been extensively tested for long-term safety, opioids remain a troubling exception. Opioid safety and efficacy studies have looked at patients using opioids for periods of 4–8 weeks. How does this inform the risks and efficacy of prescription opioids in a person taking them for 1 year? Or 5 years?

This chapter provides an overview of the known risks associated with long-term use of prescription opioids. Knowing your risks will help you make an informed choice about whether you are comfortable with opioids being part of your chronic pain treatment plan.

In addition to understanding your general risks, you must talk with your doctor about *your specific risks*. If you decide to take opioids—or if you are already on them—you should be prepared to monitor for signs and symptoms and thereby minimize your risks. Knowing and monitoring your risks also allows you to decide if the benefits of opioids outweigh the costs.

Women have greater risks than men because they are more likely to have chronic pain and therefore have greater pain treatment needs. Furthermore, pain in women tends to be more intense and to last longer than in men. Some studies show that women are more likely to be prescribed opioids and at higher doses than men. As a result, women are more at risk for experiencing the problems that come from long-term opioid use. And, as you will learn, prescription opioids can cause unique problems in women.

The following sections provide information on opioid risks according to various categories:

- Risks for All Adults
- Specific Risks for Men (see page 45)
- Specific Risks for Women of Childbearing Age (see page 46)
- Specific Risks for Older Women and Men (see page 49)

Risks for All Adults

Accidental overdose. See Unintentional overdose.

Addiction. Addiction is a risk for *anyone* when taking opioids for chronic pain. In the early days of opioid marketing for chronic pain, up until about 2005, the propaganda lore was that addiction risk associated with long-term opioid use was minimal to none. In fact, this is false. Opioid abuse and addiction are very real risks, even for people who have no history of substance abuse or addiction. Research shows that you may be at greater risk for opioid abuse and addiction risk if any of the following apply to your situation:

- Current alcohol or substance abuse
- Current cigarette smoker
- Current depression

- Current anxiety disorder (e.g., PTSD, panic disorder)
- History of alcohol or substance abuse

It is especially risky to use opioids if you have any of these factors, in part because they actually *worsen* pain* and therefore set you up for a cycle of needing more opioid medication. And, as with most of these substance abuse or emotional issues, the existence of these factors in your life just sets you up for opioid misuse.

Anxiety. Anxiety is a common experience for people who have chronic pain. If you have an anxiety disorder, you are more likely to develop a chronic pain condition because of the effect anxiety has on the nervous system. At least 30 percent of people with chronic pain have an anxiety disorder.[15] If you have chronic pain and a diagnosed anxiety disorder, you are much more likely to be prescribed opioids than someone who has the same amount of pain but does not have an anxiety disorder.

For instance, people with posttraumatic stress disorder (PTSD) are more than 2.5 times as likely to be prescribed opioids for chronic pain as are people without PTSD.† Similarly, people with panic disorder are 6 times more likely to be prescribed opioids than are people with chronic pain who do not have panic disorder. These results suggest that, in part, opioids are medicating the underlying anxiety symptoms. This is dangerous because opioids **are not approved to treat anxiety or other psychiatric issues,** *and doing so only encourages chemical coping and addiction.*

To be clear, prescribers do not knowingly write inappropriate opioid prescriptions to treat PTSD or panic disorder. But this is often

---

*Having a remote history of substance abuse does not necessarily prime a person to experience heightened pain. However, prior history of substance abuse is very strongly related to abuse of precription opioids. For this reason, opioids should not be prescribed to people with substance abuse histories.

†This is true even when studies control for the fact that people with chronic pain and PTSD may have greater physical trauma than people with chronic pain who do not have PTSD.

what happens under the surface, without anyone knowing it—and it serves to underscore the importance of evaluating and treating pain from a multidisciplinary, holistic perspective. A far better approach is to aggressively treat any underlying anxiety and to avoid opioids to every extent possible.

If you have an anxiety disorder, you also have greater risks associated with the use of prescribed opioids. For instance, PTSD is a risk factor for prescription opioid addiction and for fatal opioid overdose, particularly for US veterans returning from combat with PTSD and chronic pain. I cannot overstate this point: It is crucial that the psychological factors are treated first. And, ideally, opioids are avoided altogether if you have any of these high-risk factors.

Brain risks. Imaging research conducted at the Systems Neuroscience and Pain Laboratory at Stanford University showed that people with chronic pain who took prescription opioids for as little as 30 days showed reductions in brain volume in the amygdala region as well as alterations in other regions of the brain. After 30 days, participants stopped taking opioids and then had a follow-up brain scan after a 4-month opioid washout period. The follow-up scans did not show brain volume normalization, thus suggesting that even as little as 30 days of opioid use appears to have a lasting effect on the brain.[16]

The data clearly showed that the brain is changed by opioids, but what the brain changes actually mean is less clear. We don't know what changes mean in the daily lives of people who take opioids. And we don't know who is most at risk to have brain changes with opioid use. At Stanford, follow-up studies are currently under way to answer these important questions. For now, a global take-home message is never to assume that the medicine you are prescribed will have no lasting or negative consequences on your body: we simply don't know for sure.

Cardiac risks. Long QT syndrome is a heart rhythm disorder that involves erratic and fast heartbeats and creates risk for seizure and sudden death. Long QT syndrome can develop over time from taking methadone, buprenorphine, and high-dose oxycodone.[17] Women of childbearing age using opioids have greater risk for developing long QT syndrome than men.[18] Long QT syndrome is an indicator for ventricular tachyarrhythmias like torsades de pointes and is a risk factor for sudden death. Long QT interval is a problem that develops over time as a result of chronic use of opioids. Ask your doctor whether you need to be monitored for this condition. Everyone taking high-dose oxycodone or *any* dose of methadone should be screened regularly for long QT with electrocardiogram (ECG)—especially women of childbearing age.

Constipation. Constipation is one of the most common side effects of opioid use. It can be severe, painful, and even debilitating for some people. Stool softeners such as senna or MiraLAX are often recommended for opioid-related constipation. Talk to your doctor to see if there are other things you can do to help the problem. Focusing on proper diet, daily exercise, and drinking lots of water may reduce opioid constipation and help you avoid having to take yet another pill. Opioid-related constipation is one reason that opioids are generally not recommended for people with irritable bowel disease or other similar gastrointestinal problems, as they may simply make the problem worse.

Death. See Unintentional overdose.

Dependence. Clinical "opioid dependence" involves the melding of psychological and physiological dependence, and the term is used interchangeably with addiction. Withdrawal symptoms are typical in opioid dependence when opioids are removed. These symptoms include a mixture of physical, observable signs and psychological components linked to the withdrawal experience.[11,19] The World Health Organization (WHO) and DSM-IV-TR* clinical guidelines require

---

*DSM-IV-TR: Diagnostic and Statistical Manual of Mental Disorders, version IV, produced by the American Psychological Association. Dependence is a psychological disorder classified by the DSM.

that three or more of the following six characteristic features be experienced or exhibited:

1. A strong desire or sense of compulsion to take the drug

2. Difficulties in controlling drug-taking behavior in terms of its onset, termination, or levels of use

3. A physiological withdrawal state when drug use is stopped or reduced, as evidenced by the characteristic withdrawal syndrome for the substance, or the use of the same (or a closely related) substance with the intention of relieving or avoiding withdrawal symptoms

4. Evidence of tolerance, such that increased doses of the drug are required in order to achieve effects originally produced by lower doses

5. Progressive neglect of alternative pleasures or interests either because of drug use or due to the increased amount of time necessary to obtain or take the drug or to recover from its effects

6. Persisting with drug use despite clear evidence of overtly harmful consequences, such as harm to the liver, depressive mood states, or impairment of cognitive functioning[20]

Depression. Research shows that depression and opioids often go hand in hand with chronic pain. People with chronic pain who are also depressed are more likely to be prescribed opioids and to remain on them long term than those who are not depressed.[21–24]

The question is whether depression leads to opioid prescription or vice versa: Does long-term opioid use cause depression? It may work both ways. One study of people with chronic pain found that those who take opioids regularly have a higher occurrence of depression compared with those who do not take opioids.[21] And when researchers followed the study participants 10 years later, they found that the people who were still taking opioids were more likely to be depressed than those who were not taking opioids.[21] It is important to note that this finding was correlative; the study did not show that taking opioids for years causes depression.

To be sure, depression is associated with greater pain severity, and this increases the likelihood for opioid prescription. The proven link between depression and opioids suggests an additional risk for polypharmacy* because of the need to address both the depression and the pain.[11] The link between depression and opioid use is especially relevant for women because, compared to men, women are more likely to experience pain and depression and to experience both conditions at the same time. However, it is known that long-term opioid use disrupts sleep and hormones, both of which contribute to depression.

The human brain naturally produces opioids (called endogenous opioids). Your natural brain opioids are involved in the brain's reward and reinforcement circuitry. The release of your natural opioids provides you with pleasure following certain behaviors such as eating or sexual intercourse. Pleasure is rewarding—it makes us want to do the same behavior again to re-create the pleasurable experience. The reward system of the human brain is altered when opioids are taken long term, and this may have implications for changes in behavior, mood, and the development of depression.[25]

New research from Stanford has shown that patients who stopped opioids during an inpatient stay at the Stanford Comprehensive

---

*Polypharmacy (poly = many; pharmacy = prescription drugs) is the concurrent use of multiple pharmaceuticals. In the case of depression and chronic pain, people are more likely to be prescribed opioids and antidepressants.

Interdisciplinary Pain Program* experienced immediate and lasting improvement in depressive symptoms. Moreover, the Stanford researchers found that patients who underwent the greatest reduction of opioids had the most improvement in depression scores.[26] Patients were followed up at home 3 months later, and they reported that their moods were still improved.

Difficulty finding a prescriber. For a variety of reasons, patients taking opioids may need to find a new physician to prescribe their opioids. For example, their former physician may retire or move to another area. Patients are often dismayed and surprised to find it is not easy to find a new prescriber. Worse, some patients taking opioids have reported being dumped or abandoned by their physicians.† Doctors who are not pain specialists may not wish to manage the "complex" nature of chronic pain opioid prescribing because often the prescriptions are endless—thus leading to endless issues to be managed. Furthermore, many general physicians may feel uncomfortable prescribing opioids long term because they are not pain physicians and lack the specialty training.

Physicians also face personal risks from prescribing, including chronic pain patients misusing and abusing their prescription—and even patient death. Physicians in several states have faced wrongful death lawsuits and the loss of their medical license, thus leading some to conclude that the personal risks are too great to justify prescribing opioids. Physicians or clinics may state outright that they do not prescribe opioids,

---

*The Stanford Comprehensive Interdisciplinary Pain Program (SCIPP) is an inpatient program for people with chronic pain, most of whom seek to decrease or eliminate opioids while manging pain and withdrawal symptoms. Pain physicians, pain psychologists, physical therapists, occupational therapists, and nurses work collaboratively to maximize patients' functioning during their stay. Patients receive pain education and acquire pain coping skills as components of their pain psychology treatment. Although duration of treatment is individualized, SCIPP treatment typically ranges between 7 and10 days.

†Discussed by Dr. Steven Passik at the 2013 PainWeek conference in September in Las Vegas, NV.

thus leaving opioid-taking patients with fewer options. So-called opioid refugees have been known to resort to seeking care in neighboring states because they cannot find a prescriber in their home states.*

Driving risks. It is dangerous to drive while taking prescription opioids. Opioids may impair your ability to think clearly, and your reaction time may be slowed. Many—perhaps all—opioid pill bottles warn about the risks and caution against driving or operating heavy machinery while taking the medication. Have your physician *and* a family member weigh in on how you are thinking and reacting when taking opioids. It is important to ask the opinion of others. Discuss whether you need to plan your life so as not to require driving. I have worked with many overmedicated clients who had very poor awareness about how impaired they were, and this is exactly the point. By definition, cognitive impairment means that your thinking and judgment are off, and you risk making false determinations of your safety to drive. Many an overmedicated client has sat in my office, and the signs are unmistakable: drowsiness, slowed speech, slowed thinking, slowed reaction times.[10] If you take opioids, ***never*** drive if you have any of these signs and symptoms. If you feel dizzy, fatigued, or foggy headed, do not drive. It is not worth the risk of a motor vehicle accident, injury to yourself and others, and a charge of driving under the influence (DUI).

Drug-drug interactions. Dangerous opioid drug-drug interactions include benzodiazepines and barbiturates (see Unintentional Overdose). If you are taking opioids, you are probably taking other medicines and therefore have risk for drug interactions. Opioids may interact with other drugs you are taking. Review your current medications with your doctor before taking opioids or before starting new prescriptions. Please note that Table 3.1 is not exhaustive. **Rather, the list highlights commonly prescribed medications that impact how opioids work and therefore**

---

*www.americannewsreport.com/nationalpainreport/opioid-refugees-keynote-topic-painweek-8821537.html.

Table 3.1   Medications Require Caution If Taking Opioids

Generic Name	Brand Name	Use/Type of Medication
Alprazolam Clonazepam Diazepam Lorazepam Temazepam	Xanax Klonopin Valium Ativan Restoril	Benzodiazepines are generally prescribed to treat anxiety and sleep problems
Fluoxetine	Prozac	Antidepressant (SSRI)*
Bupropion	Wellbutrin, Zyban	Antidepressant (atypical) also prescribed for smoking cessation
Duloxetine	Cymbalta	Antidepressant (SNRI)†; also prescribed to treat chronic pain
Venlafaxine	Effexor	Antidepressant (SNRI)†; also prescribed to treat chronic pain
Paroxetine	Paxil	Prescribed to treat anxiety and depression. It is an SSRI.
Sertraline	Zoloft	Prescribed to treat anxiety and depression. It is an SSRI.
Nortriptyline	Pamelor	Antidepressant (tricyclic)
Verapamil	Calan, Isoptin, Erelan	Treats high blood pressure, cardiac arrhythmia
Cimetidine	Tagamet	Antacid
Ketoconazole	Nizoral	Anti-fungal agent
Voriconzazole	Vfend	Anti-fungal agent
Fluconzazole	Diflucan	Anti-fungal agent

*SSRI: Selective Serotonin Reuptake Inhibitor
†SNRI: Selective Serotonin Norepinephrine Reuptake Inhibitor

caution should be used if you taking opioids. The medications listed in Table 3.1 either increase the effects of certain opioids—thus increasing your risks for various side effects—or they may weaken the effect of certain opioids, and thus may contribute to opioid dose escalation (which also increases your risks). Talk with your doctor about your prescriptions and your specific risks. Also be aware that certain supplements such as St. John's Wort and Kava and grapefruit juice require caution when taking opioids because they can also affect how opioids work.

Risks for drug interactions increase when people are getting medications from different doctors. AVOID THIS. To reduce your risk, keep all your prescriptions consolidated with *one* doctor. If you absolutely must receive prescriptions from different doctors, make sure that each prescriber is aware of your current medications and doses. To further reduce your risk, always remind your medical providers of your opioid prescription *and dose* before you accept any new prescriptions. Ask your doctor directly if any new drugs you are being prescribed may have an interaction with opioids.

Emotional numbing. Some people describe feeling emotionally blunted or numb while taking prescription opioids. This can present as a reduced ability to experience joy and delight.* It can also mean a person may be less likely to experience anger—an emotion that may usefully signal that a personal boundary has been violated—and thus may enable a person to remain in situations they would not otherwise tolerate. There is a fine line between "chemical coping," or "addiction," and the effects of opioids enabling a person to, say, remain in a bad marriage. I have seen people in clinic who were not addicted, who were taking their opioids as prescribed, and their opioids caused emotional blunting that made their questionable circumstances less bothersome.

Job/employment. Be aware that if your employer drug-tests and you are taking prescription opioids, you will need to disclose information about your prescription. On occasion, medical use of opioids may pose employment problems, depending upon the job and the company policy.

---

*A reduced ability to experience joy may owe to the fact that prescription opioids alter the balance of naturally occurring opioids and reward circuitry in the brain.

Lack of benefit/worsening pain. Many people stop opioids very early on because of either lack of benefit or side effects. Opioid studies follow patients 2 months or less after they begin opioids—a honeymoon period. During this honeymoon period, the average patient reports up to 30 percent pain reduction.[9] Bear in mind that these figures offer a very early snapshot in time. Pain relief will likely diminish over time as tolerance develops. Overall, existing data often call into question the benefit of opioids for chronic pain. For the following conditions, the data more strongly argue *against* use of opioids:

- **Low back pain.** For the benefits of opioids to outweigh the risks, you should experience improved function, which means that you are able to do more of the things that are important to you. Studies of people with low back pain have found that long-term opioids do not significantly improve pain or function.[27] On average there is no solid evidence that long-term opioids are effective treatment for low back pain.[8] Instead, treatments such as exercise and cognitive behavioral therapy are shown to improve low back pain outcomes.[28–30]

- **Irritable Bowel Disorder (IBD)** sometimes called irritable bowel syndrome (IBS). Quite simply, there is no evidence to show long-term opioids are good treatment for IBD pain. Opioids reduce gut motility and, as with constipation, may further irritate IBD.[31]

- **Musculoskeletal pain.** Some researchers have argued that long-term opioids may prolong or worsen musculoskeletal pain and therefore should be avoided.[32]

- **Migraine.** Only two major open-label studies have looked at opioids for migraine. The first study was done approximately 10 years ago and recommended long-term opioids for *select* patients. However, the more recent study done at the same center found that long-term opioids provided *no benefit*, and in fact opioids appeared to make migraine *more resistant* to treatment.[33] And the largest epidemiological study to date found that people who used opioids for migraine had an increase in medication overuse headache, commonly referred to as "rebound headaches."

Dr. Sheena Aurora, migraine specialist, explains that her brain imaging research shows that a specific area of the brain— the periaqueductal gray—is abnormal in people with migraine. This area of the brain is rich with opioid receptors. Researchers believe these abnormalities make people with migraine more vulnerable to opioids. Dr. Aurora noted that other research supports this thinking. "Clinic studies show that patients with episodic migraine who are given opioids are more likely to have their migraines become *chronic*."*

Like most pain conditions, interdisciplinary care is best for migraine management. Dr. Aurora offers a specific three-pronged approach for treating migraine:

A Abortive medications (nonopioid)

B Biobehavioral approaches

C Consider prevention

Abortive medications are given to stop a migraine once it has started and are often in the triptan class of medications. Triptans allow for a targeted approach and minimize nonspecific pain medications that are associated with medication overuse headaches.

Most migraineurs can benefit from focusing on *biobehavioral approaches*, including the avoidance of triggers (i.e., caffeine, certain foods, poor sleep, and stress). Patients can also benefit from stress relaxation techniques and biofeedback. Consistent sleep,

---

*Dr. Sheena Aurora, personal communication, October 20, 2013. Bottom line: Opioids worsen migraine—avoid them.

meal, and exercise schedules also seem to reduce migraines. In particular, avoid stackable triggers, such as eating trigger foods when stressed. For some patients, migraine triggers include the timing of their menstrual cycle and chocolate. Avoiding chocolate around the vulnerable period may fend off a migraine attack.

If using abortives and employing biobehavioral strategies do not work, *consider prevention*. The addition of preventive drugs to your regimen may be imperative if headaches occur on average more than 2 days a week or, despite appropriate therapy, the attacks interfere with usual activities. The FDA has approved certain nonopioid medications for episodic migraine and one for chronic migraine. Talk to your doctor to learn more.

• **Fibromyalgia.** There is no evidence that opioids are helpful for fibromyalgia pain, and there is some evidence that suggests *opioids may worsen fibromyalgia symptoms.*[32,34–38] For this reason, opioids are not recommended for fibromyalgia pain. People with fibromyalgia may have other pain problems, such as specific neck, knee, or shoulder pain, and may take opioids to treat that problem. Bear in mind that, regardless of the reason you take them, opioids may negatively impact your fibromyalgia. If you have fibromyalgia, it is best to avoid opioids altogether.

Opioids appear to worsen migraine, fibromyalgia symptoms, and irritable bowel disorder/syndrome.

Methadone risks. Methadone may be prescribed for pain because it works on specific opioid receptors, is low-cost, and is a long-acting drug. A long-acting drug may be desirable in some cases, but it lends serious risk for overdose death because the medication remains in the body so long. Methadone has the longest half-life of opioids*—between 10 and 60 hours depending on the formulation—and this makes it easy to accidentally overdose. A person may have forgotten when they took their last dose, and taking another pill may prove fatal. A person may falsely assume that because their last dose of methadone was taken a day or longer ago that the medication has cleared from their system: not so. Methadone can remain in your body for days. Or, a person may take their methadone as prescribed and take an additional dose of a sedative—it's the combination of these medications that can be deadly. Methadone deaths typically happen because a person is taking a sedative or barbiturate at the same time, and this causes respiration and the central nervous system to slow. People simply stop breathing and die.

Reduce your methadone risks:

1. Avoid methadone if possible.

2. If methadone is under consideration, receive an evaluation from a pain physician first, as they are best qualified to evaluate, prescribe, and monitor this medication (see "What Is a Pain Physician?" on pages 34 and 35).

3. **Methadone combined with a sedative, barbiturate, or benzodiazepine can be deadly.** It is safest never to take these medications together. If you have been prescribed these medications in combination, I urge you to discuss this with your doctor to either learn why you are a specific exception to the rule or to change your prescription regimen.

4. Carefully review all medications with your doctor to ensure you are not at risk for a drug-drug interaction.

5. Talk with your doctor if you have had a recent respiratory (lung) infection, compromised breathing, or sleep apnea. In each case you

---

*Half-life is the amount of time it takes for 50 percent of a medication dose to clear from the body.

What Is a Pain Physician?

❖ A pain medicine (PM) physician provides specialized assessment and care for people in pain. Typically, a PM physician has completed a pain medicine fellowship involving extra training beyond their medical degree training and original specialty training. Most, but not all, PM physicians enter this subspecialty training through the fields of anesthesiology, physical medicine and rehab, neurology, or psychiatry. It is important to note that any physician can identify themselves as a pain physician; however, only someone who has gone through a PM fellowship and completed a certification exam can refer to themselves as a "board-certified pain medicine physician."

❖ This distinction is important since the field of pain medicine is still relatively new and encompasses a wide variety of experiences and training. Many physicians who call themselves pain physicians have only superficial training and expertise. Finding someone who has the particular training to care for your needs helps guarantee the quality of assessment and care for your problem.

❖ Pain medicine physicians often work exclusively with patients experiencing pain. The benefits of working with a pain physician means that you receive a detailed assessment and treatment plan specific to your type of pain. You are also evaluated for nonmedication pain treatments, and potentially receive multidisciplinary pain care. All initial visits with a PM physician should begin with a detailed history and physician examination. Your PM physician may order additional tests or consults to get a more comprehensive understanding of your pain problem and how it has impacted your medical, physical, psychological, and social health.

❖ Pain treatments vary based on the type of pain, among other factors. PM physicians have expertise regarding which classes of medications are best suited for each type of pain and pain condition. Many of the medications that are used for pain were originally developed for other purposes, but subsequently were found to be useful for the treatment of pain. For instance, Joe's doctor might suggest a medication such as gabapentin (Neurontin), which was originally developed to treat seizures but is actually a better nerve pain medication than an antiseizure medication. Joe might also be prescribed a medication that is classified as both an antidepressant and a pain medication, such as duloxetine (Cymbalta). Remember that while you may be prescribed a medication originally developed for seizures or depression or another condition, that medication may have great benefit for your pain.

❖ Pain physicians are also trained in other types of pain treatments, such as procedural interventions. A pain physician can determine if you are a candidate for pain treatments that do not involve pills, such as epidural steroid injections, facet injections, nerve injections, or neurostimulation (also called spinal cord stimulation). It should be noted that the primary goal of these interventions is not necessarily to cure or fix your problem. Sometimes these procedures can cure your pain. Most often the goal is to reduce your pain so that you can improve your physical and psychological conditioning and gain more control over your pain.

❖ Many pain physicians practice in a multidisciplinary pain clinic (or a pain center that integrates training providers while also doing research on pain) that offers multiple treatment approaches, such as pain psychology, physical therapy, acupuncture, and occupational therapy. Researchers have shown that chronic pain is best treated in a multidisciplinary fashion.[80] This makes sense because, if your pain is treated holistically, there is a better chance you won't simply be handed a prescription. Multidisciplinary pain care is superior to medical treatment alone in terms of improving your pain, function, and mood, and for helping people to return to work and need fewer medical visits[80]. While multidisciplinary pain clinics are often more associated with larger academic programs, there are a growing number in this community of practice. If your pain problem is of long-standing duration and you have already seen multiple physicians without improvement, you would probably benefit from being evaluated and treated at a multidisciplinary pain clinic. See page 207 in the Resources section to learn how to locate the closest multidisciplinary pain clinic.

What Is Neurostimulation?

❖ Neurostimulation is a specialized pain intervention performed by a pain physician or neurosurgeon. Its primary purpose is to reduce the frequency, duration, and intensity of pain. Neurostimulation is an FDA-approved therapy for management of chronic pain in the back, neck, arms, or legs that has been recommended by doctors for over 40 years to manage chronic pain and improve quality of life.

❖ Neurostimulation therapy is covered by many major health insurance plans, including Medicare, as well as workers' compensation programs. It carries none of the common risks associated with opioids, such as hormonal disruption, cognitive effects, sleep disturbance, and addiction. While every patient responds differently to neurostimulation, many patients are able to decrease the number of pain pills they take each day or remove them from their treatment plan completely after this therapy.

❖ Neurostimulation is a chronic pain management option that works by intercepting pain signals before they reach the brain. To accomplish this, a small device is implanted in the body. When turned on, this implanted system sends pleasant, mild electrical pulses to nerves along the spinal cord, diminishing the feeling of pain and providing what some patients describe as a massaging sensation or, in some cases, simply the absence of pain.

❖ A neurostimulation system typically consists of three components that are designed to work together to help manage pain: a generator (also called a stimulator), leads, and a programmer that allows the patient to control the stimulation. The generator is a small device, similar to a pacemaker, which sends pulses to the leads. Generators are available with rechargeable and nonrechargeable batteries. They are usually placed in the abdomen or buttock area. Leads are thin wires that deliver pulses from the generator to nerves along the spinal cord. Leads are placed in an area along the spinal column called the epidural space. The programmer is an external, handheld device, similar to a remote control, that lets a patient adjust and manage how the stimulation feels.

are not breathing well already, and methadone can compromise your breathing further and lead to risk of death.

6. You may be switched from one opioid medication to methadone—this is known as a *conversion*, and it is a very high-risk time because it is easy for dosage mistakes to be made. Many methadone deaths have occurred when patients were being converted from a different opioid to methadone. In the event that the decision is made to convert an opioid prescription to methadone, ask your doctor to discuss your conversion dose and to have it double-checked. Be sure to discuss all of your concerns with your doctor. Your life may depend on it.

Reduced preventive care. Some research suggests that basic medical care, such as colonoscopy, PAP smears, flu shots, and mammography, may be neglected in people taking opioids long term.[39] It is believed that this can happen because medical visits are consumed with issues related to opioids and chronic pain. If you take opioids, be mindful to discuss other health care issues and preventive care when you see your doctor, even if these issues are not your most pressing problems.

Sleep problems. As previously discussed, research shows that prescription opioids disrupt normal sleep cycles, your so-called sleep architecture.[40] As a result, opioids prevent people from reaching stage 4 sleep—the restorative sleep stage. People often take opioids to help with nighttime pain so they can sleep better. Opioids may help you *fall* asleep, but paradoxically they may prevent you from achieving the most restful, restorative stages of sleep. Poor sleep quality increases fatigue and next-day pain, and it is associated with greater systemic inflammation.

Sleep apnea. Long-term opioid use is associated with obstructive sleep apnea, and opioids can cause central sleep apnea.[41–45] Simply stopping opioids may cure central sleep apnea.[46,47] Sleep apnea carries many other health risks and therefore should be treated in the event that stopping opioids is impossible. In terms of pain management, it is vitally important to treat sleep apnea because poor sleep results in more pain and systemic inflammation, and may lead to a greater need for pain medication.

Smoking. If you are a smoker, the single most important thing you can do to reduce your pain is to stop smoking. Smokers have greater pain intensity than nonsmokers. Smokers also report that their pain interferes more with their daily activities. There are several reasons why smoking worsens pain. Some research suggests that smoking may suppress the body's ability to respond to stress,* and this may lead to heightened pain perception. Smokers may have greater neurodegeneration and higher levels of systemic inflammation, two other factors that may account for increased pain. The increased pain caused by smoking may lead to a greater need for pain medication.

Taking opioids may be a particularly futile strategy for smokers because smoking reduces the effectiveness of opioids. In part, this may be because smoking appears to alter the way opioids are metabolized in the body.† Researchers at the Mayo Clinic compared the effects of hydrocodone on both smokers and nonsmokers with back pain. They found that despite the smokers having used more hydrocodone tablets, they continued to report greater pain than nonsmokers using less opioid medication. Moreover, even though smokers took higher doses of hydrocodone, they had lower hydrocodone levels in their blood.[48] The authors speculated that substances in cigarette smoke (polycyclic aromatic hydrocarbons) altered morphine metabolism by activating P450 enzymes.

If you smoke, you will gain less pain relief from opioids than a nonsmoker. Smokers tend to take much higher doses of opioids without better outcomes. To the contrary, smokers have worse outcomes. Among people with chronic pain, opioid users are more than

---

*Smoking may cause dysregulation of the hypothalamic pituitary adrenal (HPA) axis.

†This is known as pharmacokinetics.

twice as likely to be smokers than are nonopioid users.[49] Smoking may contribute to dose escalation because smokers have more pain and require larger opioid doses to manage the same amount of pain compared to nonsmokers. Smoking leads to worse outcomes for pain and for people taking opioids.[49-53] For example, researchers at the Mayo Clinic found that smokers with fibromyalgia missed more days of work and reported worse sleep, greater anxiety, greater depression, greater stiffness, and greater fatigue compared to nonsmokers with fibromyalgia.[54]

Smoking worsens pain.

Smoking reduces the effectiveness of opioids.

If you smoke, the best way to reduce your pain and reduce your need for opioids is to STOP SMOKING.

Smoking makes pain worse in part because it contributes to disease processes, such as deterioration of spinal disks, and it contributes to pain from joint conditions like arthritis. Smoking also leads to increased pain perception in the nervous system.

Some doctors simply refuse to prescribe opioids to smokers because they just don't work well in people who smoke. If pain treatment does not involve smoking cessation, the elephant in the room is ignored. If you smoke, avoid opioids. Instead, focus on quitting smoking, as this alone will reduce your pain; focus on nonopioid pain management options. In terms of behavioral medicine, the same skill sets that help with smoking cessation also help reduce anxiety and suffering related to pain.

Social stigma. Unfortunately, a risk that comes with use of prescription opioids is the experience of negative judgment from others in your life. Patients I work with tell stories of being judged by friends, coworkers, family members, doctors, nurses, and pharmacists, among others. You may be labeled a drug seeker or an addict, despite the fact that you are taking opioids as prescribed for chronic pain. You may be viewed with suspicion by your own doctor if you report a lost or stolen prescription because these are red flags for possible opioid abuse. Many people experience little or no social stigma. However, I have known patients so weary of being falsely viewed as a drug seeker that they chose to stop taking opioids.

Theft. People taking prescription opioids are at risk for having their prescriptions stolen. You are responsible for storing opioid prescriptions in a locked safe. Avoid the mistake of assuming that your kids, grandkids, houseguests, or neighbors would never steal your pain medication. Take the safest route and assume that they *would*. Doing so may save a life.

Tolerance. Tolerance—needing more of the drug to achieve the same effect—is a risk associated with taking prescription opioids long term. Tolerance often leads to dose escalation in an attempt to regain pain relief. Higher doses of opioids increase the risk of overdose, side effects of all kinds, and developing physical dependence and addiction to the medication. Once tolerance is in place, alternatives to dose escalation include stopping opioids, focusing on nonpharmaceutical pain management, switching to a different opioid (opioid rotation or conversion), or focusing on nonopioid medications.

Travel difficulties. If you travel internationally, be prepared to notify the embassy of your destination country that you will be bringing opioid medication with you. It may be necessary for you to carry with you a physician letter with your name, travel itinerary, name of the opioid prescription and dose, and total amount you will be carrying.[55] Opioids are illegal in some countries, and a notarized document from your doctor may be required. In some countries with strict laws, even the inadvertent breaking of rules may result in detainment or imprisonment.

Unintentional overdose. Higher opioid doses lead to greater risk for accidental overdose. Chronic pain patients who are prescribed 50–99 mg of opioids are about four times as likely to overdose as those prescribed less than 50 mg, and patients prescribed 100 mg or more are nine times more likely to overdose.[56] In addition to higher dose, overdose is more likely in those with drug abuse or alcohol use/abuse and in people taking other prescription drugs (polypharmacy). For women, accidental opioid overdose deaths have tripled since 1999. Most commonly, opioid deaths happen because opioids slow breathing,* and after loss of consciousness breathing stops altogether. In an article in *Consumer Reports*, Daniel Budnitz, MD, a medical epidemiologist and director of the Centers for Disease Control (CDC) medication safety program, stated: "It's important to be cautious with all medications, but it's especially important with opioids. These are drugs that are easy to overdose on. One high-dose pill can kill."†

Keep yourself safe:

◆ *Never* take more than your prescribed dose of opioids.

◆ *Never* drink alcohol with opioids.

Many accidental overdoses occur when opioids are taken in combination with a benzodiazepine. Opioids and benzos make for a potentially lethal combination because both classes of drugs are central nervous system depressants. Taken together, the central nervous system becomes overly depressed and breathing can slow to dangerous levels. People fall asleep, stop breathing, and die. Be aware that death can happen even at normally prescribed doses if these medications are taken together.

---

*Slowed breathing is called respiratory depression.
†www.consumerreports.org/cro/2012/04/beware-of-potent-painkillers/index.htm

Table 3.2   Benzodiazepines to Be Avoided

Drug Name	Common Brand Name
Alprazolam	Xanax
Clonazepam	Klonopin
Diazepam	Valium
Lorazepam	Ativan
Temazepam	Restoril

Table 3.2 provides a list of common benzodiazepine medications; all benzodiazepines should be avoided when taking opioids. If you choose to remain on opioids, find other ways to manage your symptoms so you can stop the benzodiazepines and stay safe. While benzodiazepines are often prescribed for anxiety or sleep, far better treatments exist—treatments that work and do not involve pills. For instance, cognitive behavioral therapy is the best anxiety treatment, can work wonders for sleep, and has virtually no health risks.

Opioids and barbiturates/benzodiazepines are a dangerous combination of medications that *can kill you.* Do not take them together unless you have had a very careful conversation with your doctor about the risks. Know how to keep yourself safe!

Using opioids to treat bad choices. This risk is discussed extensively in chapter 6. Everyone has the ability to flare their pain by making poor choices. You can *choose* to make choices that align with your body's limitations and provide good self-care. Avoid the trap of using opioids to enable decisions that ultimately are not good for you.

Using opioids to treat psychological factors and stress. Psychological stress can flare pain and lead to the need for more opioid medication. Monitor your stress level and focus on reducing the stress in your life.

(In chapters 6–8 you will learn stress management skills.) Seek professional help to best manage your stress. Understand that depression and anxiety (including panic disorder and posttraumatic stress disorder) lead to greater prescription opioid use and to higher doses of the medications.

Beth's advice: (1) Treat psychological issues first. Your pain and your need for pain treatment will diminish following successful psychological treatment. (2) Optimize nonopioid treatment (such as neuropathic medications or other nonopioid analgesics) or nonpharmaceutical care (such as exercise, massage, and acupuncture). (3) Avoid long-term opioids.

Side effects and new prescriptions. This is a massively underappreciated and understudied risk. Opioids are associated with many different reactions and side effects. For instance, a person may begin opioids and start feeling anxious. A doctor may prescribe a new pill for anxiety, perhaps Ativan or Xanax. Over time, the opioids can lead to sleep problems or to the worsening of existing sleep problems. The doctor may then order a new prescription for sleep, such as Ambien or Lunesta. Some people who take opioids may experience irritability or mood problems. Often what comes next is a prescription for an antidepressant. In each of these scenarios, a new pharmaceutical is layered on to treat a direct side effect of prescription opioids. The result is an increasingly complex medical picture as people find themselves awash in a pharmaceutical soup. Over time it becomes very difficult to determine what is being caused by the original condition or the pain, what is an opioid side effect, and what is being caused by the combination of opioids and the new medications prescribed to treat the side effects.

You can avoid this trap. If you take opioids, view every new problem and symptom with suspicion. The opioids may be causing or worsening your problem; this is true even if you have been on them for a while because some problems develop slowly over time. Talk with your doctor. If you decide to layer on more prescriptions, be aware of the associated risks and side effects of the new drug. And especially be aware of any possible interactions between the new drug and opioids. If opioids cause you anxiety, discontinue them; do not combine opioids with benzodiazepines.

Hyperalgesia. Hyperalgesia means heightened pain sensitivity. Opioid-induced hyperalgesia, means that opioids are making a person more sensitive to pain. There is controversy among professionals about whether opioid hyperalgesia actually exists. The truth is that not enough is known, and this in itself presents a risk. Even the FDA has acknowledged that studies are needed to clarify opioid risks for increasing sensitivity to pain,* as some studies have suggested.[57–61] The conclusion from these studies is that long-term opioids contribute to changes in the central nervous system that may paradoxically increase pain. One study found when people with chronic pain detoxed off of high-dose opioids, their pain was reduced.[62] Nevertheless, the data are not conclusive. If you are thinking about taking opioids or if you are taking opioids now, be aware that worsening pain *may* be a side effect. Avoid the pitfall of thinking that worse pain means you must need a higher dose!

Even though you may feel better when you take a single dose of prescribed opioids, consider that long-term opioid use could worsen your pain.

If your increased pain cannot be easily explained by your choices (e.g., overactivity) or other factors, talk to your doctor about slowing or stopping your opioids. After a successful taper, you can assess your baseline pain level and will be able to determine whether opioids were actually lessening or worsening your pain.

---

*www.fda.gov/ForConsumers/ConsumerUpdates/ucm367660.htm (accessed September 10, 2013).

Specific Risks for Men

Testosterone and estradiol. Men taking prescription opioids long term are likely to have abnormally low free and total testosterone.[63]* Signs of low testosterone include:

* Irritability
* Low libido
* Erectile dysfunction
* Lethargy
* Depression
* Weakness

However, you may not have any obvious signs of low testosterone while taking opioids.[64] It's not enough to just go by the warning signs. Protect yourself by getting your testosterone tested, as it is the only way to know for sure. Testosterone is an important hormone that is involved in pain processing, opioid binding, maintenance of the blood-brain barrier, regulation of the neurotransmitters dopamine and norepinephrine, and maintenance of bone and muscle mass. Low testosterone impairs healing and is a source of inflammation.† *Everyone taking opioids long term should have their testosterone tested—even women.* You may wish to stop opioids to restore testosterone to its pre-opioid levels. If opioids are absolutely unavoidable as treatment, testosterone replacement should be considered and used as indicated. Any symptoms of low testosterone should abate once testosterone levels are restored. Symptoms that persist after testosterone has normalized are

---

*Between 50 and 75 percent of men taking prescription opioids have low free and total testosterone.[24] www.practicalpainmanagement.com/treatments/hormone-therapy/testosterone-replacement-chronic-pain -patients.

†www.practicalpainmanagement.com/treatments/hormone-therapy/testosterone-replacement-chronic-pain-patients

probably not the result of low testosterone and are likely from another cause such as depression.

It is often thought that testosterone is a male hormone and estrogen is a female hormone. In reality, both men and women have both hormones, though the normal amounts of each hormone certainly vary based on whether a person is male or female. Men taking prescription opioids have been found to have abnormally low levels of the main estrogen, estradiol; this is not a good thing.[63] Consider having your estradiol tested as well, and talk to your doctor about what your results mean.

Risks Specific to Women of Childbearing Age

Breast-feeding. Some women have a genotype that makes them rapidly metabolize codeine into morphine.* The CYP2D6 genotype, as it is called, will make morphine available to your breast-feeding baby and is a risk for overdose and death.[64]

Drugs taken while breast-feeding will transfer to your baby in varying amounts. To minimize risk you may talk with your doctor about the following points:

1. Start with the nonopioid medications. NSAIDs are included in this group. Be aware of NSAID contraindications and adverse effects: risks of GI and renal problems, increased bleeding, and so on. Acetaminophen may be a wonderful option in this scenario since it lacks many of the NSAID adverse effects.

2. When pain is not resolved with nonopioid medication, you must move up the ladder. If you need an opioid and you are concerned about the possible fast codeine metabolizers, use a different opioid—there is a long list of options besides codeine.

3. Remember that taking less of any drug will minimize your baby's risks.

---

*This is the P450 2D6 (CYP2D6) genotype.

Very little is known about the risks to breast-feeding infants whose mothers are taking long-term opioids for chronic pain, because to date there are no studies describing the risks. Related studies suggest that there are likely to be breast-feeding risks. Minimize your infant's risks by avoiding postpartum opioids if you can, or at a minimum avoid an increase in any regularly scheduled opioid dose during the nursing period.[65] Breast-feeding mothers taking opioids should watch infants closely for signs of opioid toxicity,[66–70] including lethargy, difficulty breast-feeding, and loss of consciousness. If you are breast-feeding and taking opioids, be sure to talk with your doctor about your baby's risks.

Infertility/Loss of Menstrual Cycle. Opioid use can reduce fertility while taking the prescription and perhaps for a period of time afterward. One study found that 52 percent of women aged 30–50 taking opioids long term lost their menstrual cycle (amenorrhea), compared to 20 percent of women with chronic pain not taking opioids.[71] This is largely due to lower levels of two key hormones involved in menstruation: luteinizing hormone and follicular stimulating hormone.* The study found that for women taking opioids their average levels of luteinizing hormone and follicular stimulating hormones were 70–73 percent lower than women not taking opioids. Other research echoes these findings.[72] Theoretically, hormones and menses should normalize when opioids are stopped. Women attempting pregnancy should avoid opioids because they reduce fertility and also because of risks for birth defects in the first trimester (see Neonatal Risks/Birth Defects).

Hormones. In addition to being at risk for reduced fertility, women have other hormonal risks, known as endocrinopathy. Studies show that women aged 18–44 who take opioids long term have low total and free testosterone, estradiol, dehydroepiandrosterone sulfate (DHEAS),

---

*Luteinizing hormone and follicular stimulating hormone are both produced in the pituitary gland.

luteinizing hormone, and follicular stimulating hormone.[71] Hormones are linked to many different systems in the body. Low hormones caused by opioids can contribute to sleep problems, depressed mood, low sex drive (libido), more inflammation, and greater pain. Academic readers and readers who are interested in the technical aspects of hormones and opioids are referred to Vuong and colleagues' (2010) excellent comprehensive review on this topic.[73]

If you are taking opioids long term, ask your physician to test your free testosterone, estradiol, and DHEAS levels to ensure they are normal. If they are not normal, you may wish to either stop opioids or talk with your doctor about a supplement plan.

Neonatal Risks/Birth Defects. For pregnant mothers taking opioids, there is a modest increased relative risk for rare birth defects for the developing fetus.[74] For example, maternal prescription opioid use increases the risk of the rare heart birth defect hypoplastic left heart syndrome from 2.4 per 10,000 live births to 5.8 per 10,000—a 2.4-fold increase that translates into a 0.06 percent chance.[74]

Researchers at the Centers for Disease Control examined birth defects in the children of 454 women who took prescribed opioids for pain related to surgery, infections, or chronic conditions between the month prior to pregnancy and the first trimester (3 months after conception).[74] They compared birth defect rates of prescription opioid–using mothers to mothers not taking opioids and found that thr risk in opioid-using mothers was between 1.8- and 2.7-fold greater. Increased risk was found for a number of heart defects, including

- Conoventricular septal defect
- Atrioventricular septal defect
- Atrial septal defect
- Hypoplastic left heart syndrome
- Tetralogy of Fallot
- Pulmonary valve stenosis

Mothers' use of opioids was also linked to a twofold increased risk for noncardiac birth defects, including spina bifida and gastroschisis. When the researchers tightened the window of opioid exposure to the month prior to conception and up to 2 months after conception, the connection between opioids and birth defects strengthened. This strengthening of the association lends greater confidence that the opioids caused the birth defects. The risk for hypoplastic left heart syndrome—a condition strongly linked to infant mortality[75]—increased 3.7-fold.[74]

Specific Risks for Older Women and Men

Delirium. Older adults are at risk for becoming delirious while taking opioids. Delirium is a temporary change in mental status that is often distressing, and it places the elderly patient at risk for accidents, falls, and related injuries. Older adults taking opioids and their caregivers should be aware that patients may experience sudden confusion and disorientation. Delirium is a sign that opioids should be stopped or at minimum that the dose should be reduced.

Endocrinopathy. Many patients and physicians falsely assume that because hormones naturally decline as we age, older people do not need to worry about opioids causing low hormones. While postmenopausal women naturally have lower hormone levels than younger women, there are still healthy hormone ranges for every age. Opioids lower hormones in women aged 50–70 *beyond* what would be expected—in fact, a 70% reduction compared to nonopioid-using women with chronic pain in the same age range.[71] Low estrogen and testosterone are associated with greater pain and loss of muscle and strength, and greater depressive symptoms are a risk owing to hormone-related changes of neurotransmitters. If you are taking opioids, you can determine your risks by getting a broad hormonal panel.

Falls/Fractures. Numerous studies have shown that seniors who take opioids are at risk for falls, fractures, hospitalization, and death related to fall complications.[76–78] Particularly in elderly patients, opioids may cause or worsen balance problems, reduce muscle strength, reduce coordination, or cause dizziness or delirium—all of which increase fall and fracture risk.

Prescription and Dose. Older women are most likely to be prescribed opioids and at the highest doses.[79] Higher doses of opioids increase the risk for all side effects and problems.

CHAPTER

4

Be Aware of Opioid Pitfalls

Pitfall #1: An Opioid "Trial" That Turns into Forever

A MEDICATION TRIAL IS MEANT TO BE a short test run of a new drug to see if symptoms are helped. If there are no immediate negative side effects and there is some level of pain relief, a prescription is typically continued. The problem is that opioids require a longer trial period than most drugs. Many of the potential negative side effects do not become apparent for weeks or months, so you need to wait for a period of time to gain a better understanding of your true level of pain relief, and the scope of your side effects.

Avoid the trap many people fall into—taking an indefinite prescription that is not helping! The key is to reevaluate and reevaluate regularly. Pain relief frequently diminishes over time. If you find that you are not benefiting significantly, talk with your doctor about stopping.

Pitfall #2: Continued Use of Opioids without Substantial Gain

In addition to monitoring for side effects, you also want to be sure you are monitoring whether you are functioning better with opioids. In other words, does taking opioids help you lead a more active life? While you may wish to be completely pain-free, this is generally an unrealistic goal that can set you up for failure, and may leave you feeling depressed or demoralized. Often, focusing on reducing pain is self-defeating, whereas focusing your treatment on the tangible goal of being able to increase an activity you love can actually make you happier—and more happiness naturally means less pain. Realistic activity goals might include being able to walk half a mile twice a week, or being able to go to the park with your children or grandchildren, or clean your house to your standards. Maybe you would like to get out of the house once a week to see friends, begin an exercise program, or return to work part-time. Focusing on increasing your activity and appropriate exercise can lead to lasting reductions in pain. If opioids have not helped you to lead a more engaged and active life, they should be stopped.

Regularly evaluate your level of function. On your own, continue to monitor your function over the course of weeks and months. Are you making progress? Are you meeting your activity goals? Are you taking good care of yourself? Are you doing your physical therapy or daily home exercise program? Research shows that when people focus on achieving their functional goals—rather than focusing on pain—they get better faster.

Pitfall #3: Overlooking Opioids as the Cause of New Symptoms

People often believe that chronic pain may be the cause of new symptoms. "Peter" was a patient I treated who developed extreme irritability and sleep problems. Peter's doctor thought he was depressed from living with chronic pain—a reasonable conclusion since irritability and poor sleep are two symptoms of depression. Peter was prescribed an antidepressant. However, the antidepressant did not help Peter's mood or his sleep—in fact, things were getting worse. Peter still had chronic pain, and now the antidepressant made him feel even less like himself. He felt detached from family, friends, and his life. Although his problem looked like depression, it was not. His problem was his medication.

I asked Peter when his symptoms started. His downhill slide began shortly after beginning opioids. I asked his doctor to run tests to confirm my suspicion: Peter's testosterone was low. Long-term opioids lower hormone levels in most people. Peter's irritability and sleep problems were the result of the opioids lowering his testosterone. Hormone imbalance often masquerades as depression because it causes changes in mood, sleep, and energy—all symptoms of depression that are caused by low hormones.

Peter had two options at this point: either supplement with prescription testosterone or stop the opioids and allow his body to naturally restore the balance in his testosterone and other hormones. Peter chose to do both: he began using a testosterone patch on his skin while we worked out an opioid taper plan. He chose to stop opioids and address the root cause of his symptoms, rather than just treat the opioid side effects.* It was also important for Peter to stop his antidepressant because the antidepressant was not helping his problem—it was actually creating new ones. By stopping his antidepressant, he started feeling connected to himself and others in his life, and this naturally bolstered his mood. As his testosterone increased, his sleep improved and he became less irritable.

If you receive a new prescription for opioids, be sure to check in with your doctor shortly afterward and talk about how you are feeling. After that initial check-in, you may not be scheduled to see your doctor again for several months. New problems may emerge during this time, and as in Peter's case, any new symptoms may be medication side effects.

---

*Notably, Peter did not just have a side effect. In his case the opioids were causing systemic hormonal dysregulation, the effects of which can have widespead and varied consequences throughout the human body and brain.

Protect yourself: Don't leave it to your doctor to make the connection between any new symptoms and the opioids. Chances are you will not see your doctor often enough, and your visits may not be long enough or focused enough for these issues to be addressed. Monitor yourself for side effects and investigate the possibility that prescription opioids may be the root cause. Then talk about it with your doctor.

Pitfall #4: Improper Storage and Disposal

Remember that your prescription opioids are narcotics and therefore have high street value and are a target for theft. Failure to properly secure prescription opioids is one of the factors fueling the epidemic of opioid-related overdose deaths. I have worked with several patients who had whole prescriptions stolen by houseguests, neighbors, or their teen or adult children. More commonly, a spouse or a child with substance abuse issues will steal a few pills at a time.

If you are prescribed opioids, you must ensure that your medications are secured at all times. Obviously, never leave prescriptions in the sight or reach of children. Prescriptions should be stored in a locked location such as a personal safe. Take the minimum amount of medication with you when you run errands or leave your home. Avoid the pitfall of becoming complacent and thinking that your opioid prescription bottle is just like the one with antibiotics or blood pressure medication. It is not. People are often dismayed to learn this the hard way, after their opioid prescription is stolen by a family member or neighbor—often someone they never would have worried about.

If your medication is stolen, you will be in the uncomfortable position of having to call your doctor to report what happened. You may need to file a police report before your doctor will replace your prescription. Your doctor may want to have a serious discussion with you since "lost" prescriptions are often a red flag that the person is abusing opioids by taking more than prescribed and thus running out early—or even selling the medication. And if your doctor refuses to replace the lost prescription, you may face experiencing opioid withdrawal symptoms.

Be sure to dispose of opioids properly:

- If you are unsure about proper disposal of opioids, you can either ask your current doctor or call your local police department. Many police departments have dedicated pharmaceutical dropoff options and programs specifically developed to protect the community.

- The FDA recommends that used fentanyl (Duragesic or generic patches) should be disposed of by folding the adhesive side of the patch together and flushing the patch down the toilet.* Flushing used patches prevents accidental opioid exposure and overdose deaths in young children by preventing them from finding improperly discarded patches in the trash and placing them in their mouths or sticking them on their skin.

Pitfall #5: Taking Opioids to Manage Anxiety

Most people who suffer from anxiety do not realize that they may be taking opioids in part to manage their anxiety.† All they know is: "My pain is worse and I need more medication for my pain." And they are right: their pain is worse. Most people do not understand how anxiety factors in. Their pain is worse because anxiety worsens pain. If the underlying anxiety is not treated, it can be easy to fall into this cycle:

Anxiety ⟹ Pain ⟹ Opioids

Here, the opioids are treating a consequence of anxiety: worse pain. If the anxiety were treated, pain would be reduced and there would be less need for opioids.

---

*www.fda.gov/drugs/drugsafety/ucm300747.htm (accessed October 6, 2013).

†This point is also covered in chapter 3 in the Opioid Risks section under "Anxiety"

Relying on opioids to medicate anxiety is dangerous because it can lead to addiction. Some people tell their doctor they have anxiety, and right away they are prescribed Xanax, Ativan, Valium, or some other medication. Yet even taking these medications for anxiety may undermine the goal of gaining confidence in one's ability to manage their emotional state.

The best treatment for anxiety is therapy that focuses on learning skills to help calm the mind and the body (material covered in chapters 6–8). Even severe panic can be treated with learned skills that are practiced regularly. It is vital that you learn how to be more in control of your mind and your body—this will bring down your anxiety and therefore lessen your suffering and your need for pain medication. Consider working with a pain psychologist or anxiety specialist for at least a few sessions to be sure you are best managing any anxiety you may have.

Pitfall #6: Believing You Won't Be Able to Reduce Opioid Use

Withdrawal symptoms are simply a sign that opioids have been removed from your system too quickly. If you miss a dose of regularly prescribed opioids, your body will probably let you know about it. Missing a dose of medication, stopping opioids abruptly, or lowering the dose of opioids too quickly can cause opioid withdrawal symptoms. Your body will be accustomed to having a certain amount of medication in it, and when that amount is suddenly missing, your body will react. Often withdrawal symptoms are highly distressing and even painful.

Withdrawals naturally encourage a person to retreat back to the opioids to stop the discomfort. Often people interpret withdrawal symptoms as a sign that they must remain on opioids. This is false. Everyone can successfully taper off opioids without experiencing withdrawals. The solution is to taper very slowly. Some slow tapers may take months to complete. You may need other types of support, so talk with your doctor or see an opioid taper specialist* to find out what you need to do to taper successfully.

Pitfall #7: The Indefinite Use of Opioids

The most common reason people begin an opioid prescription is for the treatment of short-term pain, known as acute pain. Consider the person who is prescribed opioids for surgery or for a severe injury. In the beginning, everyone believes the prescription will be brief, that healing will take place and the prescription stopped. But for some people, their pain does not stop even after "healing" takes place; the pain becomes chronic. Then the opioid prescriptions continue. If this scenario sounds familiar to you, be sure to talk to your doctor about other types of medications that may help your pain.

Joe was a patient who was prescribed opioids for a work-related injury that crushed his leg. He was started on opioids, and they helped him after his surgery. He healed from surgery, but his pain didn't stop. He was diagnosed with chronic neuropathic pain—the nerves in his leg were damaged. The opioid prescriptions continued because he was still having pain. But Joe had two different pain problems; one of them was helped by opioids, whereas the other was not. The opioids were good for the pain related to his surgery, but now he had a new type of pain—neuropathic pain from the damaged nerves—and opioids are not the best medication for neuropathic pain. When the opioids didn't work, he took more and more in a desperate attempt to lessen his pain. Unfortunately, he was taking more and more of the wrong medication. What Joe really needed was a nonopioid medication that best treats pain from nerve damage.

---

*A medical opioid taper specialist may be a certified pain physician or an addictionologist. A behavioral opioid taper specialist is likely to be a doctoral-level clinical psychologist who specifically works with people with chronic pain to reduce their need and use of opioids.

Avoid Joe's pitfall: Talk with your doctor about possible nonopioid options. Recall that most general physicians receive very little training in chronic pain management. If this is not an area of expertise for your doctor, or if you would like another medical opinion, ask to be referred to a pain physician. Most general physicians are happy to provide a referal for a pain specialist consulation.

Like Joe, Joan fell into the pitfall of having her pain care treatment focused solely on opioids. Even when her condition didn't improve over time, none of her caregivers considered that opioids might be causing more problems than they were helping. Joan's story also illustrates how patients can be overmedicated and still be undertreated for pain—a problem that has a surprising solution.

ò

Joan's Story

Joan is a witty 54-year-old woman with chronic pain who came to see me in clinic.* I looked forward to our sessions because she asked hard questions, wanted to get better, and knew that in order to get better things needed to change. She had lost much of her function and quality of life and was determined to get herself back. I admired her resolve.

Joan had been taking opioids for 8 years. Although the opioids were prescribed for low back pain,† she also had pain all over her body, fatigue, and a general "sick" feeling that constitutes fibromyalgia, a syndrome involving widespread muscle pain.

Her primary care physician was unhappy. The opioids were not working well, the dose kept escalating, and new pains kept emerging. Now Joan was contending with frustration from her prescribing physician, and she was feeling judged. Tears streamed down her face as she sat in my office.

"I don't understand it," she half-sobbed out of exasperation. "I feel like I'm being treated like a drug seeker. I don't want the drugs! I just

---

*Joan wished to tell her story anonymously; her real name and details of her story have been changed to maintain patient confidentiality.

†It is now known that opioids are not a good treatment for low back pain.

want the pain to go away. I went to my doctor for help with my pain and she prescribed me oxycodone. Now everyone acts as though I'm doing something wrong."

ə∾ ᖇ

She was right, of course. Hers was a story I heard every day.

The reality is that Joan, like many other pain patients, was set up to look like a drug seeker because the opioids were not taking away her pain as everyone expected them to. I explain to patients that the very term "painkiller" is misleading and a misnomer, given that opioids are known to basically "take the edge off" pain; but very rarely do they render chronic pain patients "pain-free." If a patient tells their doctor a drug isn't working, the doctor may very well prescribe more of it. This is one reason opioid doses escalate.

Another reason doses escalate is that the body develops tolerance to an opioid dose over time. Tolerance is a natural, inevitable physiological consequence that every patient experiences. It is not the same as abuse or addiction.

Yet tolerance may be viewed with suspicion. Does the patient really "need" more medication,* or are they liking it too much? Are they gaming the system? Until someone reaches the outer edges of normal behavior, it is difficult to know.

Pitfall #8: The Blame Game

When opioids do not work well, patients may end up feeling blamed for it. They may ask for more medication because that's the only "solution" that has ever been offered to them. Like Joan, most people do

---

*The term "need" is subjective, and this is why treating pain is more complicated than other conditions. Undoubtedly, there is a need for the patient to have their pain and distress better managed. However, to assume that a patient needs more opioid medication is a dangerous simplification of the issue and a major reason the problems with opioids—and the so-called epidemic—exist in the U.S. today.

not want more opioids; they want less pain. Asking for medication may be perceived as "drug seeking." For someone struggling to manage life with chronic pain, adding shame on top of suffering may be intolerable. Chronic pain is already a condition that tends to be viewed with skepticism; after all, you can't see someone else's pain. Sufferers may feel judged by their families, friends, employers, and insurance companies. They hope the people they turn to for medical help will be compassionate.

Avoid the blame game pitfall:

1. **Look beyond opioids.** Ideally opioids are avoided, but if they are prescribed and necessary, never rely on opioids alone for pain control. Use the methods in this book and seek multidisciplinary pain treatment.

2. **Have an up-front agreement.** You and your doctor will both benefit from having an up-front agreement: If opioids are not improving your life and enabling you to do more things than before, you and your doctor both agree to stop the medication and look to alternatives—without assigning judgment or blaming one another. In doing so, you will be freed from feeling the blame of being labeled a drug seeker, and your doctor will be freed from being judged as unwilling to treat your pain or withholding pain care from you. In truth, good patient care means stopping what is not working.

Tim's story illustrates many opioid pitfalls as well as the benefit of working with a pain physician and a pain psychologist in a multidisciplinary pain center. When he began receiving specialized pain care, many of his problems improved—even those that seemed unrelated to his pain.

ה‌ב‍ ‌ב‍ה

Tim's Story

Usually a physician will refer patients to me in the pain clinic, but Tim Roberts went to his doctor and asked for a referral to see me. He was profoundly depressed. A year and a half before, he had been in a serious motorcycle accident. As he told me his story, I recalled reading about his accident in the newspaper right after it happened.

In the summer of 2010 Tim was riding his motorcycle with a group of other motorcyclists on Interstate 5 near Wilsonville, Oregon. The car ahead of him came to a sudden stop, forcing him to lay his bike down on the pavement at 60 miles an hour. He skidded on his back across the multiple highway lanes. He was fortunate to not be run over by any other vehicles but sustained major injuries in the accident, including spine trauma.

Tim looked the part of the typical Harley-Davidson rider when I met him. He wore the signature menacing wardrobe of a tough guy—including Doc Martens boots—and his large frame was accented by a long black goatee and a requisite number of tattoos and body piercings. Based on his appearance alone one might guess that he lived as hard as he looked, but nothing could be further from the truth. He was an insightful and intelligent blue-collar worker with minimal formal education who did not drink, take drugs, or use profanity, and he was a strong believer in strict family values.

It was clear when I met Tim that he urgently needed help. He was taking high doses of opioids. He had severe irritability and he suspected the opioids were causing him to be depressed, but he didn't know what else to do to cope with his pain. So he came to me to help him get off opioids and reclaim his life.

Since irritability is one of the signs of low testosterone caused by opioid use, I asked Tim to have his doctor test his testosterone as a first step. Once this was condition was confirmed, Tim and I began to work together over the next 2 months to reduce his opioid use, along with the use of other medications. Our sessions mirror the actions presented in this book in chapters 6–10. What follows is a more detailed account of how Tim left his opioid use behind.

We first reduced his opioids and other pharmaceuticals. Then we treated the problems caused by the opioids. By using this combined approach, Tim improved dramatically. He regained control of his life and his depression, and thoughts of suicide remitted. His sleep improved, and he started taking care of himself. He got out of bed each day, ate regularly, and began feeling like himself. He still had chronic back pain—even severe pain at times—but no longer was he suicidal, depressed, exhausted, irritable, and vegetative.

Over the course of our 2 months of meetings, Tim developed a personal empowerment plan (chapter 10), and he used the information I gave him—the same information in this book—to successfully taper off opioids. Tim is happy to have himself back, even if he still has pain. The truth is, he always had back pain even with all the medications. Now his life is working, and so are his relationships.

ॐ ॐ

Tim found that by stopping what wasn't working—and by getting the right care—he improved his life. Good chronic pain care involves a multidisciplinary approach. Multidisciplinary pain treatment will help you either avoid opioids or get off them while still mitigating your pain.

Some multidisciplinary programs are intensive, meaning that participants attend day programs consisting of physical therapy, pain psychology, occupational therapy, and the like. A study of a 3-week intensive multidisciplinary pain treatment program for chronic low back pain—which included weaning off of and stopping opioids—showed that the program reduced participants' pain and depression and improved their activity levels.[80]

Another study looked at 600 veterans with moderate to severe chronic pain who completed a pain rehabilitation program. At

In Tim's Words

Tim wanted to share his story, hoping that it might help others struggling with pain and opioids. He talks about his motorcycle accident and how he came to be prescribed opioids in the first place.

"I broke my L4 and L5 vertebrae and fractured my S1, resulting in a laminectomy and diskectomy over the course of three operations. The first operation was plagued with mistakes made by the doctor, resulting in an emergency surgery to remove and repair the mistakes. So I was in really bad shape for about 18 months. And that brings us to the opioid pain relief treatment. Just a note, prior to all these pain pills, I didn't even drink beer! I was sober, no drugs or alcohol, and here I sit, nearly 2 years into my adventure . . . dependent on pain pills."

Tim acknowledged that his opioids were very helpful in the beginning. Over time, however, the opioids became more a daily routine, and he was gaining little or no relief at all. He found he was taking them for *"maintenance purposes"* only—mainly to prevent withdrawal symptoms.

Given all of Tim's surgeries and complications, he found he had an open-ended amount of pills made available to him. An exit strategy was never discussed because his doctors focused only on the moment at hand. "I was obviously in a great deal of pain, so my doctor saw it best to keep my medicine levels fairly high to incorporate the maximum amount of pain relief. Unfortunately, once you go up so high in your dose, it's hard to bring it down."

But he needed to bring his opioids down because his insomnia was severe, and his sleep quality was worsened by the opioids.

"I had a complete inability to get any meaningful rest at all. Then depression," he said. *"Some people really do need opioids,"* Tim advises others in his situation, *"but I would say be careful. I wish I had done things differently, and I wish the doctors had other options for me outside a handful of pills. It just seems so typical of today's medical services . . . just take a pill."*

admission, some veterans were taking opioids and some were not. Veterans who were taking opioids were weaned off of them, and afterward everyone received the same multidisciplinary treatment program. The researchers found that the veterans who stopped taking opioids benefited as much or more from the pain program as did the veterans who were not on opioids.[81]

One small study showed that 90 percent of patients who were detoxed off high-dose,* long-term opioids had their pain lessen.[62]Notably, this study included people who wished to stop their opioids because they felt they were not helping their pain.

Studies show that patients benefit from stopping opioids when they receive intensive multidisciplinary pain care.

Pitfall #9: Opioids May Worsen Pain

There are many reasons why stopping opioids may help your pain. Animal studies show that opioids cause the animal to be more sensitive to pain—this is known as hyperalgesia.[86–88] Pain clinicians and researchers are divided on whether opioids cause hyperalgesia in humans.[57,58,61,82] The human studies are not conclusive. Some researchers believe that the pain reductions many patients report after stopping opioids is evidence that opioids worsen pain in people.[62] In 2013 the FDA called for more research into the opioid risks of developing increasing sensitivity to pain.†

---

*Between 45 and 450 morphine equivalents daily, with most patients in the range of 150–250 mg.

†www.fda.gov/ForConsumers/ConsumerUpdates/ucm367660.htm (accessed September 10, 2013).

A potential pitfall of long-term opioids is that they may actually worsen your pain by causing greater sensitivity to pain and the development of new pain problems.

For an average person taking opioids long term, the opioids become less effective over time. It is difficult to know whether this is because of tolerance or because a person develops pain sensitivity from the opioids. In an article on the topic,[32] pain expert and researcher Dr. Leslie Crofford explains the distinction between tolerance and hyperalgesia:

Patients who are opioid tolerant should have no increase in baseline pain sensitivity but require an increased dose of opioids over time to achieve the same analgesia reached with a lower dose. Patients with opioid hyperalgesia have increased pain sensitivity. Distinguishing tolerance from hyperalgesia in an individual patient might require clinical demonstration of reduced pain sensitivity after opioid detoxification.

In other words, you cannot know whether your body is getting "used to" opioids or whether the opioids are actually causing the pain to become worse. In either case you are set up to need higher doses of opioids.

In addition to hyperalgesia, animals given opioids also are more sensitive to stress and have greater levels of inflammation in their blood.[89–91*] Inflammation is a reaction from the immune system. It can be caused from injury, illness, and other kinds of physical stress, and also from psychological stress. Inflammation is linked to various diseases and to the development of chronic pain.[92,93] Inflammation worsens pain, so it

---

*Cytokines—a marker of inflammation— are also measured in the cerebrospinal fluid.

is important to avoid things that cause inflammation.[89,94] While animal studies clearly show that opioids cause inflammation, human studies are less conclusive.

Pitfall #10: Being Overmedicated and Undertreated

Many opioid prescriptions are written in cases where opioids are poor treatment for a specific pain condition. For example, Joan was prescribed opioids for fibromyalgia and for low back pain—two conditions that do not benefit from opioids.[32,37] Her pain worsened as she continued taking opioids, and this led to her being prescribed higher and higher doses.

At her peak dosage, Joan was taking 210 mg of opioids each day: 40 mg OxyContin ER TID (extended-release formula, taken three times daily for a total of 120 mg), 30 mg of OxyContin IR TID (immediate-release formula, taken three times daily for a total of 90 mg).

Joan was prescribed what's called "round-the-clock" opioids, meaning that the 8-hour extended-release formula she was taking three times daily ensured that opioids were in her system 24 hours a day. She was also prescribed extra opioids on top of that—immediate release—for what doctors call "breakthrough" pain—pain that she might feel despite having the round-the-clock opioids in her system.

When I asked Joan if the opioids helped her, she paused before responding. "In the long run they hurt; in the short run they helped. When I was first put on them, I was in excruciating pain and there weren't other options made available to me. I admit it was a relief when the culture changed and people wanted to treat pain. The problem was that, regardless of the intent, the treatment harmed in the long run. And no one looked long enough to stop it."

Like most patients, Joan felt she was not informed of the long-term complications. She spent years living with memory problems, cognitive haziness, severe fatigue, severe pain, and difficulty performing activities like standing, walking, and lifting. She also had depression and severe sleep deprivation. When I met her, it was clear that she was highly dysfunctional and overmedicated. Ironically, Joan was overmedicated and undertreated at the same time—she was being given high doses of the wrong medicines.

Over time Joan had become depressed, which compounded all her symptoms, including her pain, and fueled a cycle of adding prescriptions to treat her worsening problems. The extra medications were not helping her, and she began to suspect they were actually contributing to her deterioration.

I worked with Joan over the next few months to help her meet her goals of getting off opioids and off sleep medication. I recommended a very slow taper for Joan, especially given her anxiety about the taper and her fear about experiencing a "pain rebound" when stopping the opioids. Five months after beginning her slow opioid taper, she was down to 20 mg of OxyContin per day with a goal of being completely off the medications within the following weeks.

What happened next shocked her but did not shock me because I had seen it many times before: She got better.* She was able to do more than before. Her mood improved. Her sleep improved. She told me that she got her brain back and could think clearly. She felt like she had returned to herself, and once again, she was right.

"It has never been clear to me how much of my depression in the past 8 years has been because of the opioids. For me, the most soul-destroying aspect was losing my intellectual capacity—they robbed me of my memory and my sharp thinking. That was a large part of my personal identity. My memory was shot to hell, I couldn't think, and I was dead tired all the

---

*Joan's experience is not uncommon—many people discover reduced pain following opioid taper. Baron and McDonald provide some empirical support for this clinical observation and individual patient report.[62]

time because I also was sleeping so poorly. And I never got better—I got worse. At my highest doses of opioids, my pain scores were never better than they were before. Now that I'm almost off the opioids, my pain is so much better. I didn't sleep well for years—the whole time I was on the opioids. I was barely sleeping, and that fed the pain."

Joan's story illustrates some of the complexity of prescribing opioids for chronic pain. A patient visits their physician in excruciating pain. What does a good doctor do? They try to treat the pain and alleviate suffering with whatever means are available.

Like many patients, Joan wished that opioid risks and side effects were monitored and alternative treatment options discussed with her on the front end. She never had the chance to discuss the connection between her medical problems and her opioids. She wished she had been told that opioids worsen fibromyalgia symptoms.[32,36,37,95] Had she known about the risks, she could have been looking for problems and steering the conversation in the right direction during her medical visits.

"Follow-up doctor visits are flawed because the focus is on what is happening right now, and we get stuck dealing with the pain of the moment versus the big picture. The big picture being: *Are these drugs even helping?* Has anything changed since they were first prescribed? What are good alternatives?"

Joan paused and smiled ruefully.

"But then the other problem about alternatives is that even if patients have access to them, their insurance probably won't pay for it. You can't get body work covered. If you are poor—and most people who are disabled with chronic pain are poor—you don't have the resources or access to nondrug options. Even finding you—I was lucky. Most people do not get to see you or someone who does the work you do, either because of insurance issues or because they don't have local resources. The meds are their only option."

Joan hit on a major flaw in the current health care system. Indeed, there is a great need to improve patient access to pain education and to comprehensive pain care that includes alternatives to opioids and other pharmaceuticals.

After being on opioids for so long, Joan had no idea what her real pain "baseline" was—her nonopioid pain level. Like most people, she feared going off opioids because she thought her pain would be much worse. And, in fact, if withdrawals are experienced, then pain *will* worsen temporarily, long enough and severe enough for most people to retreat back to opioids. Many people cannot tolerate withdrawal pain and falsely believe that it will be permanent. Joan learned that when she tapered her opioids slowly enough she avoided withdrawals, remained comfortable, and was happy to discover she had *less* pain.

I asked Joan whether there was a clear point at which the opioids were no longer helpful.

"I don't know, it sneaks up over time," she answered. "The pain remained and even seemed to get worse, so my dose was increased. No alternatives were presented to me. Now I think the pain was worsening *because* of the opioids. I do know for sure that the pain has improved since I've gone down on the opioids, and my side effects are improving too."

When asked what she would say to someone with chronic pain who was considering taking opioids, she replied that she would want to hand them a big cautionary note. "I would want everyone to know clearly and up front how it would affect their memory and sleep and other systems, and to know what else they could do to help their pain besides taking opioids, and that it's important to take as little of them as possible."

She paused. "It took me 10 years to find you.* It took 10 *years* before I had alternatives come through the system, alternatives that helped me stop the medication cycle. Part of the trap is that, as a patient, it's hard to problem-solve your way out of the mess and see the larger picture for yourself because you can't *think* right. A lot needs to change in the

---

*Joan had chronic pain for 2 years before she was prescribed opioids.

system." Joan is right. We must help people make informed decisions about their pain care and help them get access to alternative treatments that have lasting results.

Pitfall #11: Balancing Policing versus Patient Care

Joan's medical team monitored her opioid use with urine drug screens. Drug screens are done for two reasons. First, prescribers want to make sure patients are not taking illicit drugs, like cocaine. Generally, state and national guidelines require or strongly recommend that doctors give a urine drug screen for *all* patients prescribed opioids—so it does not automatically mean your doctor is suspicious of you. Urine drug screens protect the public because they can help identify people who are most likely to sell their prescription on the street.

Urine drug screens can confirm whether the prescribed opioid is actually in a patient's system—as it should be. If the urine screen comes back negative for opioids, the doctor has good initial evidence that their patient may be selling their opioid prescription, a practice known as "diversion." Drug tests are necessary because of the subepidemic of people selling prescription opioids, whether obtained for a true medical condition or whether the "patient" lied about having pain in order to get and sell the opioids.* And there is an epidemic of opioid death tragedies that happen when people take an illegal OxyContin or other opioid with alcohol, not understanding that the combination is deadly. People drift off to sleep under the sedation of opioids and alcohol and their breathing slows, then stops. They simply don't wake up.

Opioid death is also a risk for people taking the prescription for chronic pain.

Higher doses of opioids create greater risk for unintentional overdose death. Quite simply, take too much opioid medication, take

---

*Lying for the purpose of secondary gain is known as malingering. In this case, malingering to obtain a narcotic prescription is illegal and prosecutable.

opioids with alcohol or with other prescribed drugs that also depress the central nervous system and slow your breathing, and you can die. The death toll has mounted in recent years.

It may be rightly argued that policing is part of good patient care. If a doctor discovers a patient taking opioids is also using cocaine, they may steer the patient to addiction treatment and harm reduction. Beyond patient care, discovering and stopping opioid diversion keeps prescription opioids off the street, makes the community safer, and may save lives.

Nonetheless, doctors may focus on monitoring for the abuse or criminal misuse of opioids and fail to monitor for the most important patient care issue: Are the opioids actually *helping*? Are there any harms?* In Joan's case, she was drug-screened on every visit to ensure she was compliant with her care, but she was not being monitored carefully for her *response* to opioids. And in fact her response was poor: overall, the opioids helped her pain a bit in the beginning, but as her initial pain relief diminished, many new problems took root and flourished.

It's not that physicians *want* to police opioids. After all, doctors are not in the business of law enforcement. Doctors are required to comply with laws set forth by state and national agencies. The laws are good for the community but in reality may do little to improve chronic pain care. A focus on improving access to pain care would be the most effective solution to the opioid problem. Many advocates focus on the issues of addiction and "doctor shopping," the recreational and criminal use of prescription opioids—major problems that have contributed to the overall "opioid epidemic" in the United States. But for chronic pain, the biggest problems are that opioids alone are inadequate and that doctors and patients alike do not have access to good pain care. Policy makers might be surprised to discover that everyone's goals

---

*A harm caused by an opioid is known as an iatrogenic effect: an unintentional problem caused by the treatment itself.

would be met if patients had access to effective pain treatment—treatments that are already proven to provide lasting benefits!

With better pain treatment, fewer patients will begin opioids, and more patients taking opioids will need less of them, thus preventing opioid dose escalation. As long as the focus remains on medications alone, patients who take opioids are at risk for opioid dose increase. Consider three main reasons opioid doses escalate:

1. Opioids may not provide pain relief.

2. Even if opioids work well initially, over time tolerance develops and more opioid is needed.

3. Opioid side effects may lead to greater pain and more medication. For instance, opioids often lower hormone levels and disrupt sleep, thus leading to greater pain. More pain = more opioids.

Avoid the pitfall of assuming that a higher opioid dose will be better for your pain.

Assuming that a higher dose will improve your pain is a trap fueled by having false expectations about opioid pain relief. More is not better. People may think "if I take more, it will work just like it did that first day I took the medication." However, scientific studies tell us that the pain relief from opioids is limited and that it diminishes over time.

Have realistic expectations about opioid pain relief. In general, taking higher doses does not gain you a better result—just more and worse side effects. Instead of dose escalation, use the techniques in this book and focus on nonopioid pain control strategies to augment or substitute for opioids.

Yvonne's story* further illustrates how increasing opioids when they are not working can lead to more problems.

≈   ≈

Yvonne's Story

Neither I nor any other clinician would have told Yvonne to get off opioids. She had every reason and medical indication to be taking them. Even her primary care physician believed she should remain on opioids. Yet my experience working with her reminded me that even in the case of catastrophic injury, patients can get off opioids if they are motivated—and they may have good reasons why they want to.

In 2007 I was a pain psychologist at Oregon Health & Science University. One morning I picked up the newspaper from the driveway, poured a cup of coffee, and took a few minutes to read the front page before heading in to the pain clinic. I froze as I read the article on the front page. The story described a horrible tragedy.

A local woman had spent the afternoon swimming with her 16-year-old son and granddaughter. They left the pool and were loading items into the trunk of her car when a speeding truck came from behind, pinning the woman against her vehicle at her knees and crushing her legs almost entirely off her body. Her son screamed in horror. She was in shock as the driver reversed his truck, dragging her body 20 feet along the curb, scraping off skin and infecting her wounds with debris. An ambulance took her to the hospital where both of her legs were amputated. This woman's story brought me to tears as I stood in my kitchen. I wanted to help her, but we had no connection.

Two and a half years later I was working a normal clinic day in the pain clinic. A new patient was on my schedule that afternoon. I went

---

*Confidentiality is sacred in the psychologist-client bond, and case details are never disclosed without explicit consent from the client. Yvonne offered to include her story in this book. She provided permission for the details of her medical history, her psychological history, and her direct quotations to be published, for the specific purpose of helping other people with chronic pain avoid some of the problems she encountered.

out to the waiting room to greet her. She was beautiful: long dark hair, friendly eyes, and a warm smile. She was in a wheelchair, a double amputee. "Hi, I'm Yvonne," she said.

Once seated in my office she began to tell me her incredible and tragic story. "Did I read about you in the newspaper in 2007?" I asked her. "Yes," she replied. "That was me on the front page."

She paused and took a breath. "I have been looking for you for two and a half years." Then she added, "I want off the opioids."

She had been prescribed opioids for postsurgical pain following her amputations, and the prescriptions never stopped. She had chronic amputation-related pain in the stumps of her limbs, back pain from being wheelchair bound, and pain in her wrists from overusing them to push herself in the wheelchair. She determined that her opioid medication was causing more problems than it was helping. Her sleep was a mess, and she was having trouble with memory and concentration. She felt they were also making her apathetic toward her rehabilitation goals in physical therapy. Her other side effects included constipation, poor appetite, withdrawal symptoms, trouble swallowing, rash, and clumsiness.

"My doctor thinks I'm crazy to try, nobody thinks I can do it, but I am determined," she said with steely resolve. And then, she looked at me: "I need your help."

I knew I could help Yvonne because she was fed up and willing to work for results. Getting off opioids and managing pain without medications does take work—and not everyone is willing to do it. But Yvonne had her sleeves rolled up.

Psychologists tend to hear it all, so it's not often that we are surprised by what our clients tell us. Yvonne managed to surprise me. In fact, I found myself stunned as she told me her whole story.

It turned out that the man who hit her was taking opioids for back pain related to a previous car crash he was involved in.* In fact, he was

---

*It is unclear whether the opioids he was taking at the time of the accident were for acute pain or chronic pain.

on a cocktail of prescription medications that included antidepressants and muscle relaxants in addition to his opioids. On the day of Yvonne's accident, he had been sent home from his job at an auto parts store 4 hours before his shift ended because he was incapacitated and unable to run the cash register. He lost control of his vehicle on the drive home and crashed into Yvonne. It was a tragic irony that in a split second Yvonne was suddenly caught in the opioid painkiller trap.

In the beginning, opioids were a critical part of Yvonne's medical care plan, as might be expected after such a harrowing ordeal. "I had 18 surgeries over approximately 2 months," she told me. "I was sedated in an induced coma for 21 days; once I was awake, I was given high doses of morphine through an IV for about 10 more days."

Then, as she began to heal, her IV was stopped and she was given shots of morphine instead, a change Yvonne didn't like since she didn't like the way she felt when she was given the drug. Unfortunately, without the morphine shots Yvonne began to feel anxious, so she requested anxiety medicine; Ativan (a highly addictive antianxiety medication) was added to a list of 22 medications she was taking. One of those drugs was time-scheduled oxycodone, and she was required to sign a statement upon leaving the hospital that she would take those medicines as prescribed.

Months later, as she was being fitted with prosthetic legs, Yvonne began to realize the opioids contributed to multiple issues. She was told by her doctor to slightly increase her dose before fittings in order to handle the pain of fittings and learning to walk. She found that the medication caused her to feel woozy and unsteady on her feet, which made the whole process more difficult instead of easier.

She also had severe sleep problems. And her pain was worsened in two ways. First, she had chronic constipation that was very painful. Second, an hour before she was due to dose her opioids, she would experience withdrawal symptoms that included extreme pain. Yvonne said she began to wonder, "Was this how much pain I was really in, or was it a 'rebound' effect of withdrawal?"

Her doctor tried to resolve the problems by increasing her opioids. Extended-release morphine was prescribed, with oxycodone to be used in between for breakthrough pain. Unfortunately, this made the condition much worse. "I became caught in a world dominated by nausea, pain, anxiety, and withdrawal symptoms," Yvonne told me." Eventually, that plan was stopped.

Yvonne's opioid use also impacted her life in other ways. For instance, she ran into problems when she needed to visit the emergency room on several occasions (ironically, due to constipation caused by the opioids she was taking). "On more than one occasion I was treated as a drug seeker," she said. "It was assumed I was there to beg for more medicine. The truth was I had access to all the pain medicine I wanted or needed from my personal physician."

She was also viewed suspiciously at her primary care facility when she met with doctors who were not familiar with her case. One doctor grabbed her bottle of drugs, dumped the contents onto the exam table, and started counting the pills using his bare, unwashed hands. When the count revealed she was telling the truth about the number of pills she had, the doctor offered no apology. "I never wanted to be on opioids less than that day, when I realized I would have to place those pills in my mouth," Yvonne said.

❧　❧

Like Tim, Yvonne benefited greatly from opioids to treat the trauma from her accident and also after her surgery. In the long run, however, opioids complicated her rehabilitation and her quality of life. Yvonne was able to taper off opioids by applying the information you will learn in the next five chapters.

Part II

Your Solution Is to Gain Control

CHAPTER

5

Know and Treat the *Full* Definition of Pain

I OFTEN HEAR PATIENTS SAY, "I don't want the opioids, but I don't know how I can get through the day without them." They are afraid their pain will only worsen without the opioids. My response to them is this:

I will teach you a program, and if you invest yourself in it, your suffering will lessen, and you will find you naturally "need" less pain medication. Reducing your pain and suffering requires work on your part, but you will keep for the rest of your life the knowledge and skills you gain. You can learn how to need less pain medication. The journey to self-empowerment is slower than taking a pill, but it works better. No doctors needed, no prescription required. The first step is to begin treating the entire experience of pain, as it is defined.

What Is Pain?

Everyone has felt pain. You know it when you feel it, though you may not have thought much about how pain is defined.

The Merriam-Webster Dictionary[96] defines pain as follows:

---

pain **1:** a state of physical, emotional, or mental lack of well-being or physical, emotional, or mental uneasiness that ranges from mild discomfort or dull distress to acute, often unbearable agony, may be generalized or localized, and is the consequence of being injured or hurt physically or mentally or of some derangement of or lack of equilibrium in the physical or mental functions (as through disease), and that usually produces a reaction of wanting to avoid, escape, or destroy the causative factor and its effects. **2:** a basic bodily sensation that is induced by a noxious stimulus, is received by naked nerve endings, is characterized by physical discomfort (as pricking, throbbing, or aching), and typically leads to evasive action

---

Merriam-Webster refers to pain as being either physical or emotional. While physical and emotional pain can occur at the same time, these definitions seem to place the physical and emotional into separate categories or types of pain. An example of emotional pain would be grief, while an example of physical pain would be pain experienced from a broken foot. Separate categories.

And yet, it turns out that even physical pain is more than just the sensory "ouch" felt in the body. The International Association for the Study of Pain (IASP), a global professional organization for pain research, treatment, education, and policy with more than 8,000 members in 129 countries, defines pain as follows: an unpleasant sensory* and emotional experience associated with actual or potential tissue damage, or described in terms of such damage.

Now let's focus on the important part of the definition.

Physical and emotional pain are no longer in separate categories. Pain is both a sensory and an emotional experience. According to the IASP, *psychology is built into the very definition of pain.* A basic principle

---

*"Sensory" means what you feel in your body; the physical sensation of "hurt".

of psychology holds that how you feel is strongly influenced by how you think. This is a critical point: your thoughts shape how you feel physically and how you feel emotionally. Understanding the power of your mind will help you gain control over your experience of pain.

Pain is an unpleasant sensory *and emotional* experience.

Because the experience of pain involves your thoughts and emotions, it's easy to see how you could find trouble with prescription opioids. The lines get blurred. You may end up taking more opioids to medicate your emotions, and this is a foundation for addiction. But you can run into many other problems besides addiction. Research shows that if you feel anxious or fearful about your pain, or if you have problems with anxiety, you are more likely to be prescribed opioids. Once you have the opioid prescription, you are at risk for *unwittingly* using it to medicate pain that is flared by your anxiety. All of this can be happening behind the scenes while you use your medication *exactly as prescribed*.

Among people with chronic pain, those who are depressed are three times more likely to be prescribed opioids than those who are not depressed.[24] People with an anxiety disorder may be up to six times as likely to receive opioids for chronic pain as are those without an anxiety disorder.[97]A fair question to ask is, what are opioids really treating?[98] Many prescriptions could be avoided if pain was treated for what it really is. If treatment addresses the underlying factors that feed distress and worsen pain, fewer prescriptions will be written.

You have probably been asked to rate your pain at your doctor's office. Pain is usually rated on a 0–10 scale (with 0 = no pain and 10 = worst pain imaginable); sometimes a 0–100 scale is used. Your pain rating describes the intensity of your pain experience, both the physical and the emotional parts of it. Naturally, you probably have not thought about the "emotional" part of your pain score because it's hidden inside something that's already invisible to the eye—your pain!

To better understand the emotional part of pain, think of your physical experience as being more on the surface. To use a metaphor, if you imagine that your body is like the water in the sea, your *physical* experience would be the waves on the sea's surface. Your *emotional* experience is like the currents of the sea. The currents run below the surface, are quite powerful, and often determine the height and patterns of the sea's waves.

Acknowledging the emotional aspect of your pain does not make your pain less real or any less medical. It does not mean that you are making it up or that your pain is your fault. It does not mean your pain is a psychiatric or emotional problem. Unfortunately, most people with chronic pain have heard that their pain is just "in their heads." Your pain is real and legitimate. Your pain is a medical concern that deserves treatment.

Your mind is a major asset in your pain treatment. Research shows that the mind is so powerful it can actually overcome the effect of opioid medication, something I discuss in detail in chapter 6. Opioids may have a place in your medical plan, but your true power lies in learning how to harness the power of your mind to better control your pain experience. In chapter 10 you will use this information to develop your empowerment program, and this will give you lasting control.

Pain is not something that just happens to you. You participate with your pain. Your diagnosis wasn't your choice, but the choices you make every day determine whether your pain gets better or worse. Similarly, how you think and feel determines whether your pain experience worsens or improves. As you learn about the specific ways in which you are participating with your pain, you can target those areas of your life to gain control and relief.

Your experience of pain is influenced by your thoughts, feelings, choices, stress, and beliefs. No wonder many primary care physicians feel out of their element in treating chronic pain. They are! Thoughts, beliefs, perceptions, stress, daily choices, behaviors, and emotions cannot be "fixed" with an opioid, and medical doctors are not trained in psychology. Pain psychologists—specialists with a doctoral degree in clinical psychology and advanced training in the field of pain management—are best qualified to perform these assessments.* However, there are very few pain psychologists compared to the millions of people living with chronic pain. Thus, doctors are often left to treat chronic pain while ignoring half the definition of pain and many of the factors that influence pain.

If you or your doctor do not know all the factors that influence your experience of pain, you may be set up for problems down the road. Psychological factors can lead to overprescription of opioids. And once opioids are started, patients often remain on opioids for years, placing them at risk of developing other health problems. Patients miss an opportunity to take control of their pain without opioids and are left with the negative consequences, including escalating doses that work less well over time.

This painkiller trap is avoidable. Although pain is often treated as a purely physical problem, it is in fact the most exquisite example of mind-body communication. And the communication works both ways (see Figure 5.1 on page 84). How you think affects your pain, and your pain can also affect how you think. How you feel influences your experience of pain, and your pain also influences how you feel. You may notice that your pain is worse when you are under stress. Stress worsens pain, and pain causes stress. As you well know, living with chronic pain is stressful.

There may be very clear medical reasons why you have chronic pain. Even so, these other factors determine how much you suffer

---

*Health psychologists are generally well trained in treating chronic pain.

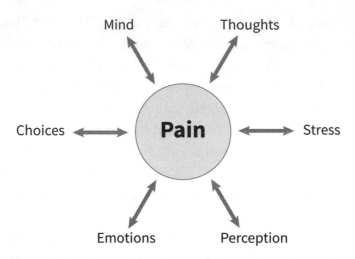

Figure 5.1 Pain is Influenced by Your Psychology, Physiology, Behavior and Environment

from pain. Consider the following with regard to how the mind influences pain:

- Although you may "feel" pain in different parts of your body, all pain is located in your brain because your brain processes pain signals from all over the body.
- Emotional pain lights up the same areas of the brain associated with physical pain.
- Research shows that beliefs and expectations are so powerful they can override the effect of newly given opioids. This means that your mind is more powerful than pain medication.
- The choices you make each day have the power to make your pain better or worse and are more important for pain control than opioids.

Pain Is in the Brain

If you break your arm, it is almost guaranteed to hurt. While you feel pain in your arm, strangely, that pain is actually located in your brain. Certainly, signals were sent from your arm to your brain, but it is the brain that interprets those signals as pain. The same is true for chronic pain. You may experience pain as being located in a specific location (e.g., your lower back) or even throughout your entire body. But the pain is really situated in your brain. This does not mean that pain is "all in your head." The fact that your brain controls pain does not make it any less real.

Without the signaling and interpretation in the brain, we would feel no pain. Using functional magnetic resonance imaging (fMRI) and single-photon emission computed tomography (SPECT) imaging, scientists and clinicians are able to produce images of brain processing under given circumstances. The processing of pain signals activates several regions of the brain, sometimes referred to as the pain neuromatrix.

Consider a broken arm. The injured arm sends signals that travel through the central nervous system to the brain. The brain registers pain. This example is quite simple, and it is only part of the story. The brain is not a passive computer that receives and registers pain signals. Instead, the brain is very active in either shrinking pain or growing pain.

You don't even need your body to feel pain—but you do need your brain. The best example of this is phantom pain, which is experienced by most amputees after they have lost all or part of an arm or leg due to injury, cancer, or another cause. Even though a person's leg was amputated, phantom pain means the person experiences pain in a part of their body that is no longer there. Phantom pain may be chronic and excruciating.

Chronic pain is a "stuckness" of the pain signaling in the central nervous system. Opioids can block or reduce the perception of pain signals, depending on whether they are taken for a short period of time or long term for chronic pain. This is where psychology enters the picture. Your thoughts and feelings have the power to amplify or soften your pain, and acknowledging their power unveils opportunities to harness the power of the brain to change your pain.

People are unwittingly using the power of their brains to make their pain *worse*.

Nobody wants more pain, yet every day people worsen their pain because they don't have the right information available to them. Susan was unwittingly worsening her pain—until she learned how to regain control.

∂ ∽

Susan's Story

In 2009 the opioid epidemic was in full swing, particularly in the state of Oregon where I was practicing. Primary care physicians were swamped with chronic pain patients requiring extra medical visits to manage pain that was not improving on opioids. Patients and doctors alike were exasperated and desperate for help—in many ways each believed the other was the problem, without understanding the role of the opioids. To address this issue, I developed and taught a 2-hour pain class that focused on how to minimize the need for opioids. I conducted the classes on occasional evenings in a family medicine clinic at Oregon Health & Science University. Class participants were referred by their doctors, most of whom were seeking guidance in how to treat these "complex" patients.

The class was an overview of the content presented in the next few chapters of this book. I taught the patients about chronic pain, why their opioids were failing them, and what they needed to do to regain control of their pain and their lives. I met Susan when she attended my pain class one evening. She was a 46-year-old high-powered attorney who had stopped practicing law to stay home and raise her three children. She had chronic pain from several medical conditions, including degeneration in her cervical spine (neck) and fibromyalgia. Staying at home seemed like a practical decision for the entire household, and as her pain increased, she was glad that she wasn't working long hours at the office.

Susan was in distress when I met her. She felt out of control and anxious and was taking Xanax for anxiety and Ambien for insomnia. She was also taking high doses of opioids for her neck and shoulder pain as well as using a fentanyl Duragesic patch.* She was in a vicious cycle: her anxiety was making her pain worse, and her pain was making her more anxious. Despite all the medication she was taking, her pain was still severe, as was her stress level at home.

"I need to gain control over my pain and my life, but I have no idea how to do this," she said. "I feel like I'm doing everything yet nothing is working." She was either pushing herself to do things in spite of her pain, or she was in bed trying to recover from a pain flare brought on by having pushed herself so hard. In either case she was struggling, and her constant struggle was sucking the joy out of her life.

Susan's pain and suffering was particularly distressing to her because she had always been in control of her life—until now. Her doctor was unhappy with all the medication she was taking, and she was viewed as a classic "problem pain patient." She had an alert placed in her medical chart to warn her medical providers that she was on a special opioid agreement—-a clear indicator of a patient who was "noncompliant" with her opioids. She wanted her life back and herself back, but she couldn't imagine getting off the opioids with such constant and severe pain.

---

*Duragesic is a brand-name transdermic patch that delivers fentanyl, a synthetic opioid, continuously through the skin.

In the class Susan learned how she was participating with her pain. She learned that in big and small ways, she had more influence over her pain than she realized. She found that she could change her pain—for better or for worse—by changing her emotions, her thoughts, and her choices.

The solution to Susan's pain

I met with Susan for private sessions every 2 weeks for several months, but such one-on-one sessions are not necessary for you since this book provides the road map you need to get the same result. However, if you want additional support, you might contact a local mental health therapist who can help you stay on your path to recovery.

છે જ

The Body. In the first session Susan learned that—like most people with chronic pain—the way she was responding to her pain and to her stress was automatic and unhelpful. She learned how to control her reactions and in doing so gained control over her experience. After years of being prescribed medications to change her levels of physical and emotional distress, Susan was surprised to learn that she could actually calm her mind and her body without a pill (you will learn how to do this, too). I gave her a pain management audio CD* and asked her to listen to it at least once daily and ideally more often than that because she had so much anxiety. By listening to the CD regularly, she was retraining her mind and body with methods proven to reduce pain and suffering. A big contributor to Susan's neck pain was the load of tension she carried in her neck muscles. Regular use of the audio CD allowed her to begin releasing her neck tension, thus reducing her pain. She learned to turn her awareness into her body and to detect what her body needed so that she could begin taking better care of it.

---

*The pain management audio CD is a 20-minute, guided relaxation. The audiofile that accompanies this book is of similar format with an added binaural component.

The Day-to-Day. Next we focused on what was happening in her daily life. She acknowledged that she did a lot for her family—too much, in fact. Her children did few, if any, chores. Susan was the household cook, chauffeur, and maid, despite the fact that her kids were fully able bodied and ages 13, 16, and 17. She had trained her children to expect her to do all the work for them. She was enmeshed with her kids and was unable to maintain good boundaries with them. She would cave in when faced with their disappointment or disapproval. She was bewildered at how she could possibly stop the cycle. "I've asked them to do more around the house, but it never happens," she lamented. Instead, she would fall back into her role as servant. This was the first thing we aimed to change.

I coached Susan to stop picking up the slack for others, literally and figuratively. She began leaving their dirty laundry piled up in their bedrooms. If they needed clean clothes, they were forced to do the wash themselves. She stopped straightening up their rooms and instead began closing their doors so their messes didn't encroach on her clean home. She stopped catering to her 16-year-old daughter's every whim—including driving her to school—and lovingly yet firmly informed her that she was to begin taking the bus. In doing so, Susan found she had time freed up for self-care, like yoga and gym exercise. She began creating independence for herself while simultaneously encouraging greater independence for her kids.

This was win-win for everyone. Sure, her kids complained, but they needed to begin taking on appropriate levels of responsibility. Susan found her family could tolerate being inconvenienced and that she could tolerate their disappointment. She stopped spending all her time and energy inappropriately catering to others. Setting firm limits with her children allowed her stress and her pain to lessen, for three reasons:

1. She learned to set appropriate limits and was no longer pushing her body so hard in an effort to please her family and reduce her own guilt. In doing so, she eliminated all the overwork that was

pushing her into greater pain levels, and she also freed up time for herself.

2. She took better care of herself and thus began meeting her own physical and emotional needs.

3. She used the relaxation response audio CD twice daily and, in doing so, she reduced her anxiety, stress, and muscle tension and was falling asleep faster.

4. As she reclaimed control over her life, she became calmer and more relaxed, and from this calm state she made better decisions. Her choices supported better pain control, and she developed confidence in her ability to manage her pain, her emotions, and her stress. Her newfound confidence allowed her to become centered and grounded within herself.

Susan's progress with pain management meant she was able to meet her goal of tapering off her medications. She stopped the Xanax first. This was the easiest. As she managed her anxiety with the steps just outlined, her need for Xanax melted away. As her pain was better managed, she began cutting down on her fentanyl Duragesic patch— literally. Each time she was placing a new patch, she took scissors and cut the patch smaller and smaller before applying it. On her own and without her doctor's knowledge, she was tapering her dosing of fentanyl by cutting her patch a bit more each time (*not recommended*).* She acknowledges it wasn't easy, but she was determined to do it, and she was determined to change her life choices to make it possible.

Along the way Susan realized how much her stress levels were linked to her opioid use. She noticed that when her daughter was being obstinate and argumentative, she would reach back to rub the

---

* **IMPORTANT: This is not a recommended technique!** Please consult your prescribing physician before making any medication changes. It is especially risky to "alter" opioid medications, such as cutting patches or chopping pills— this can change the rate at which medication is delivered into your system and may be dangerous to your health. Again, not recommended.

fentanyl patch on her shoulder. "I know now that I was instinctively trying to medicate the stress by rubbing the patch to release more medication," she said.

The Mind. Susan learned how to change her thought patterns so that she was no longer "catastrophizing" her pain. **Catastrophizing** is a term used to describe when you are thinking and feeling fearfully about pain, expecting things to get worse, worrying and feeling helpless about it, and not able to focus on much else other than the pain and how awful it is. (Catastrophizing is covered in detail in chapter 7).

Before I first met Susan, she worried about her pain getting worse, and she felt there was nothing she could do about it. She wasn't coping well mentally or emotionally, and her distress was contributing to her pain and medication use. Through treatment she learned how to keep her mind calm and how to help herself make choices that supported her primary goal: managing her own stress and pain rather than catering to others. She also learned that by taking excellent care of herself she was a great role model for her children. Before, her children were learning that it's OK for Mom to sacrifice herself—after all, she doesn't really count or deserve to be taken care of. Now, they were learning that Mom deserves to be respected and well cared for. She was teaching them by example that excellent self-care is healthy and essential. Through her actions she was modeling important, positive values that would shape their lives.

The Self. As Susan tapered off opioids, she began "feeling" more. She was surprised to feel joy at times and anger at times—healthy emotions! She acknowledged that the opioids had left her feeling somewhat numb—to physical sensation and also to her emotions. She was pleased to reconnect to a full spectrum of emotions.

Her anger turned out to be good information. It informed her that something in her life needed to be addressed. So she began addressing things directly and appropriately, and thus started nipping her stress in the bud. She developed a healthy level of assertiveness with her husband and with her kids, and while there were some growing pains, the whole family benefited. It's not healthy for anyone when a family member becomes numb and passive.

As Susan began feeling more she connected with her authentic self, she started to realize what was missing in her life. She discovered she wanted to do more outside the home in a structured way, and now that her pain was better managed, she felt ready to realize this goal.

When I last saw Susan for follow-up, she reported that her blood pressure was much lower, to the point that her cardiologist was impressed and asked what her secret was. She was excited to tell me the secret was the work we did together.

"It's really the result of all this work we've been doing in session and that I've been implementing at home—making life changes to reduce my stress and pain and to get off the prescriptions. I can't believe I have my life back," she told me.

One of the best things to come from all of Susan's progress was her surge in energy. She found she had more energy available to channel in productive ways, whether it was exercising, connecting with friends and family, doing the craftwork she loved, volunteering, or going back to work. "I was really surprised at how much energy the opioids robbed from me," she said.

Susan is inspiring. She still has her medical conditions and limitations, but she is living her best life possible. She tapered off her Xanax and Duragesic fentanyl and is now tapering off her Ambien. Instead of popping a pill to sleep, she is focusing on calming herself in the evening by turning off the TV and computer in the hour before bedtime. She is eating dinner earlier so she is not overly full at bedtime. She is listening to her relaxation audio CD before bed so that she readies her mind and her body for sleep. She is focusing on her making these changes herself so that she doesn't need to rely on the Ambien.

Taking pills may be easier on the surface, but Susan would prefer to have her life back. And she would prefer to know that she is in control of it, not a drug.

The Link between Emotions and Pain

Your emotional responses are part of your pain experience—a very important part. Think for a moment about how you feel when you experience severe pain. Often people report severe pain as being stressful, terrifying, or dreadful. Other pain responses may include helplessness, depression, anxiety, or fear.

Pain triggers an emotional response. Your emotional response helps determine whether your pain gets better or worse.

Pain is a negative sensory and emotional experience. Your emotions and your physical sensations—what you feel in your body—engage in an endless feedback loop, interacting and enhancing one another. In fact, there is less and less distinction being made between psychological and physical pain as scientific evidence continues to show how blurred the lines are between emotions and physical health.

For instance, studies show that if you feel helpless about your pain, you are less likely to recover from an injury such as whiplash.[99] Feeling helpless about pain is linked to poorer health, greater pain intensity,[100–102] and fatigue.[101]

Psychological stress activates the same regions of the brain that are associated with pain.[103] This is true for everyone, whether you are healthy or have a diagnosis of degenerative back disease, fibromyalgia, or chronic pain from cancer treatments. No matter your diagnosis or the "cause" of your pain, stress will worsen your pain. This is good news because it gives you a clear avenue to reduce your pain: by targeting your stress and emotional responses.

Emotional pain and physical pain share brain circuitry

- Social pain—feelings of social rejection or loss—activates the areas of the brain associated with physical (sensory) pain.[104–107] Social pain leads to increases in physical pain.[108]

- Physical (sensory) pain primes you to be more sensitive to social pain. The implications may be that people with chronic pain experience are more vulnerable to social stress.

- Your brain makes little distinction between physical pain and emotional pain.[108,109]

- Social stress causes greater pain sensitivity in healthy women and in women with fibromyalgia.[103*]

Emotional Hurt ⟷ Bodily Hurt

An important part of Susan's story was the fact that the stresses in her family caused her both emotional and physical pain. Only by addressing the emotional stress/pain did she gain control over her physical pain. The result was that she needed less pain medication. Like Susan, you may find that opioids dull your physical and emotional pain, thus making you less motivated to deal with the underlying issues. In doing so, the opioids help maintain problems that are ultimately causing you emotional and physical pain.

This cycle leads to reliance on medications. It is also a foundation for addiction.

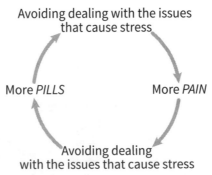

---

*This study only included women, but the findings are likely true for men as well.

Freedom from opioids requires that you deal with the issues that cause you emotional pain. Emotional pain may result from a stressful job, a divorce, past trauma, loneliness, feeling unappreciated, and so on. Discover whether you have emotional pain in your life and take serious steps to address it. Your emotional pain is as important as your physical pain, so be sure to give it the attention it deserves. Accessing support can be very helpful—and sometimes essential. Consider working with a respected therapist to help you find a pathway to relief.

You may also find emotional relief through different strategies or a combination of strategies, such as acupuncture, exercise, reiki, group support, online support, journaling, individual counseling, and the like. Experiment and find what works for you. Above all, if you have a toxic situation in your life, such as an emotionally abusive boss or an unhealthy relationship with a family member, partner, or friend, find ways to minimize your contact with the toxic person or situation. Minimizing your exposure to this stressor will provide you with emotional protection. Seek support in finding ways to protect yourself. Your emotional and physical well-being depend on it.

CHAPTER

Calm Your Nervous System to Reduce Your Need for Prescription Opioids

Out of every crisis comes the chance to be reborn

—Nena O'Neil

The Awesome Power of Your Mind

HERE ARE A FEW FACTS to consider about engaging the power of your mind to help your pain:

* Your thoughts have a powerful effect on your pain and your physical body.

* Negative thoughts and expectations are known to worsen pain, delay healing, and even override the effect of opioid medication!

* Most people are not using the power of their minds to help their pain. Instead, many people are unwittingly *worsening* their pain!

* Harnessing the power of your brain is an essential part of empowered pain control; it helps you minimize your use of opioids and other medications.

* Regularly calming your nervous system with mind-body skills reduces your suffering.

How to Change Your Pain Responses: Retrain Your Brain and Body

Pain acts as an alarm, alerting you to the presence of danger—and the need to escape the threat of harm. Consider the threat of having encountered an angry dog. If the dog were to bite you, the pain you would feel would be very useful information. The pain signals to your body to move quickly to escape further injury. In this sense, pain is protective and important to your survival.

Obviously, your behavior is motivated by the desire to stop the pain. Less obvious are the other automatic responses that happen when you feel pain. Your body automatically responds to the pain "alarm" without you even thinking about it, and often without you even knowing about it. Pain absorbs your attention, making subtler pain responses far less noticeable.

Pain acts as an alarm in your nervous system and causes the following automatic responses in your body:

1. Faster heartbeat

2. Quick and shallow breathing

3. Tightened muscles as they "brace" against pain

4. Constricted blood vessels

5. Distressing thoughts

6. Severe pain can trigger the release of cortisol (a stress hormone) and inflammatory factors into the bloodstream[110]

Automatic pain responses serve the purpose of preparing you to escape the source of your pain. In the case of a dog biting you, the pain response works because it prepares you to run to safety. Or, if you place your hand on a hot stove your pain alarm system will tell you to remove your hand quickly, to avoid severe burn. The pain response/alarm system works great in cases such as these where there is a clear threat of harm that you are able to escape. In these cases, pain responses serve their purpose and stop once the threat of harm is removed, and your nervous system returns to its natural calm state.

Chronic pain is different. How do you escape pain that coming from inside your body? You can't—and the automatic responses that are triggered by your pain alarm system are now useless because you cannot run away from your chronic pain. Rather than being helpful, your automatic pain responses actually *worsen* your chronic pain. Experienced regularly, automatic pain responses cause lasting changes in breathing patterns, muscle tension, and thought patterns—all of which increase your pain. Living with chronic pain for months and years changes your body and your nervous system.

In order to gain control over your pain, you need to retrain your mind and body to counteract the negative effects pain has on your nervous system. Pain sends a message to your nervous system that there is a need to act quickly. You will gain relief by changing the message—you will train your nervous system to remain calm. You will learn how to quiet the alarm.

It may sound strange, but a lot of the "pain solution" involves noticing what is happening in the *other* parts of your body when you are in pain, and working to change *that*.

Tune in and observe the rest of your body when you are in pain. What is your breathing like when you are in pain? Is your breathing different than it is when you are falling asleep? Are your muscles tense or relaxed? Is your mind calm? Take your heart rate and notice whether it is higher than usual.

The Connection between Pain and Stress

Think now about what you experience when something incredibly stressful happens. Imagine that you narrowly miss a car crash—slamming brakes, screeching tires, gripping the steering wheel in terror. In everyone, severe stress triggers a *stress response*.

The stress response includes the following:

1. Faster heartbeat

2. Quick and shallow breathing

3. Tight muscles

4. Constricted blood vessels

5. Distressing thoughts

6. The release of stress hormones (cortisol and adrenaline) as well as inflammatory factors into the bloodstream.[110]

The list probably looks familiar to you. Your body responds to stress exactly as it responds to pain. In fact, the pain response is a *type* of stress response. Living with chronic pain is stressful, as you can probably attest. And here we establish that **the experiences of pain and stress produce overlapping responses in the mind and body**. Both ramp up your nervous system, and this is why reducing your stress is a critical part of reducing your pain. In turn, having less pain will reduce your need for prescription opioids.

Less Stress ➤ Less Pain ➤ Fewer Opioids

The stress response has been shown to make people more sensitive to pain,[103] so reducing your stress responses can directly reduce your pain. Stress reduction is a key factor in supporting the positive changes outlined in Table 6.1, which in turn also lessen pain.

Over time chronic pain and stress cause lasting changes in your brain and in your body. Shallow breathing and the repeated tightening of your muscles can become your body's baseline default mode, such that your breathing remains shallow and your muscles remain tight even when you don't have pain. These stress-related changes become your new "normal" as your body becomes conditioned by them. Essentially, chronic pain trains your nervous system to remain on high alert. Chronic pain can cause a vicious cycle that leads to more pain.

Your adrenal glands may become exhausted from overproducing cortisol, leading to an eventual depletion. Low cortisol is associated

Table 6.1 How stress reduction leads to positive changes that lessen pain

Positive Change	Why This Positive Change Lessens Your Pain
Fewer automatic stress and pain responses	Reducing pain/stress responses calms your nervous system and helps reduce your pain.
Less muscle tension; more muscle relaxation	Tight muscles can create or worsen pain. For instance, tight neck muscles may cause tension headaches, tight back muscles can worsen or maintain back pain, etc.
Less anxiety; a calmer and clearer mind	Anxiety feeds your pain experience. You make better choices—ones that are good for pain control and overall self care—with a calm mind.
More freed-up energy	You will have more energy to do things like exercise, stretching, or physical therapy—activities that support good pain control.
Better sleep	Poor sleep leads to greater pain intensity the next day. Sleep better and you can reduce your pain.
Overall better health	Chronic stress is linked to many types of conditions and diseases, including chronic pain.
Reduced inflammation in the blood	Stress causes inflammation:[110] inflammation is associated with worse pain[111-113] and need for pain treatment.
Reduced emotional distress	When you are coping better emotionally, it is easier to deal with pain.

with worsening pain because it leads to increased inflammation throughout the body.

Quite simply, chronic pain changes your body at the muscular level, at the psychological level, and at the biochemical level. *Your body may be in a constant low-grade stress response.* Now imagine what happens when you have a pain flare on top of that.

Changing Your Pain and Stress Responses

It may seem unfair that your body automatically responds to pain and stress in a way that creates *more* pain, *more* stress, and *more* chronic disease. The good news is that you can train your mind and body to have a better response—one that helps you. It is called the *relaxation response.*

The relaxation response should be called the "health and well-being response" because it has such a powerful, positive effect. The relaxation response calms your nervous system. In a calm state, your brain is much less likely to perceive physical sensations as threatening. Essentially, your pain signaling is dampened.

The relaxation response works by canceling out your responses to pain and stress that end up worsening your pain. Just as light and dark cannot coexist in the same room, it is impossible for you to have a pain/stress response at the same time as a relaxation response. They lie at opposite ends of the continuum (see Table 6.2).

As you can see in the table, the relaxation response is the opposite of the stress response: it includes relaxed muscles, a slowed heartbeat, and nice slow and deep breathing. The relaxation response allows your blood vessels to "dilate" or open wide, so you get good blood flow throughout your body and into your hands and feet. As your blood flow improves, your hands and feet become warmer. One way to measure a relaxation response is to use a thermometer strip to measure increases in the skin temperature of your fingers. When your body relaxes, your mind also relaxes. You notice calmer thoughts and feelings when you are having a relaxation response. Research shows that the relaxation response changes your entire experience of pain.

The Relaxation Response Is a Wellness Response

The relaxation response improves the delivery of oxygen to the cells of your body, thereby reducing stress on your system. One reason why exercise is so good for health is that it opens the blood vessels and gets

Table 6.2   The Response Continuum

Pain/Stress Response	Relaxation Response
↑ Heart rate, blood pressure	↓ Heart rate, blood pressure
Quick, shallow breathing (↑ respiratory rate)	Slow, deep breathing (↓ respiratory rate)
Racing, negative thoughts	Calm, positive thoughts
Muscular tension	Relaxed muscles
Cooler hands and feet (due to ↓ blood flow)	Warmer hands and feet as blood vessels open wider and blood flow increases
Increased pain	Dampened pain
Stress hormones released (cortisol)	No cortisol increases
Inflammatory factors released in the blood	Anti-inflammatory factors released in the blood

The goal is to move this way ➡ ➡ ➡ along the continuum.

Spending more and more time in the relaxation response conditions your mind and body toward wellness and reduces suffering from pain.

good blood flow into the hands and feet; this reduces risk for vascular problems related to diabetes and other conditions. Even if you have a limited capacity for physical exercise, you can reap some of the benefits of improved blood flow by using the relaxation response often. Good blood flow to your feet, for example, improves wound healing and helps prevent skin ulcers.

By using the relaxation response, not only will you be able to quash your pain/stress response in the moment (see Table 6.3 on page 106), but with very regular practice you may recondition yourself and reduce the baseline levels of tension you hold in your body. This means that no matter what your pain level is, you will naturally carry less tension as your body adjusts into a more relaxed state of being.

Most people find that the relaxation response feels good and it is naturally rewarding to practice it. Consider that when you sigh you are deepening and relaxing your breath. When you achieve a full relaxation response, it's as if your *entire body* is sighing.

Relaxing Is Different From the Relaxation Response

It is important to know that the *relaxation response* is different from everyday relaxing. For some people, drinking a beverage while watching television is relaxing. Some may describe relaxation as the absence of work. For others it may mean knitting, or talking to a good friend, or taking a rest. When we simply relax, we may notice some of the hallmarks of the relaxation response, but *not always*. It is possible to be doing something that should be relaxing, such as having dinner with a good friend, and still have tight muscles and shallow breathing.

The relaxation response is more than just a state of enjoyment; it has measurable physiological endpoints. Take a moment to review Table 6.2. Slowed heart rate, lowered blood pressure, reduced muscular tension, warmer skin temperature (blood flow), and slowed breathing are all physiological qualities.

Sometimes people take medication to help calm their mind and their body, but medication is not necessary. In fact, it is better to calm mind and body without medication. By triggering your relaxation response on your own, you will feel (and be) more in control of your body and your experience, and this is one of the most important aspects of good pain management.

Getting to the Relaxation Response

Like pain, the relaxation response occurs in the brain. The breath provides a powerful gateway to the relaxation response and is a powerful link between your mind and body. **As the breath goes, so go the body and the brain.** As you deepen and slow your breath, your heart rate slows. Your blood vessels automatically dilate, and your muscles begin to relax. Soon you notice that your mind is calmed. By slowing and deepening your breath, you trigger an automatic wellness cascade—a full relaxation response. This is quick and powerful mind-body medicine you can do yourself—free of charge!

Two important things to know: (1) how to slow your breath; and (2) how to deepen your breath. The combination of the two—slow, deep "belly breathing"—is called **diaphragmatic breathing** because it engages the diaphragm, the main muscle involved in breathing.

The diaphragm plays a major role in the **parasympathetic nervous system,** the part of the nervous system that controls relaxation, digestion, rest, healing, healthy immune responses, and cardiovascular functions such as heart rate and blood pressure. People with chronic pain typically have overworked parasympathetic nervous systems. The **sympathetic nervous system** is responsible for defending against "attacks." Your brain automatically perceives pain as an attack, and this is what drives the stress/pain response. The "guards" are sent out: the stress hormones cortisol and adrenaline (a fight-or-flight response that helps a person run away to escape a threat), heart rate increases to prepare for escape.

When the diaphragm is engaged through the breath, signaling is sent to the brain that the muscles in the body need to relax. In this way, you do not need to focus on relaxing your muscles per se; you can simply focus on shifting into diaphragmatic breathing, and the muscular relaxation happens automatically! Diaphragmatic breathing increases oxygenation and immediately begins to reverse the stress/pain response. As you sink deeper into relaxation, you experience mental relaxation as well. As you come full circle into mental relaxation, you can see that breath is indeed the foundation of the mind-body connection.

Most people tend to breathe from high up in the chest, using only a small volume of their lungs. The problem is that short, shallow breathing helps keep tension in your muscles. Think of it this way: your muscles tend to mirror your breathing. If your breathing is tight, your muscles will be tight. If your breathing is very relaxed (slow and

Table 6.3   The Relaxation Response is Your Antidote for
Pain/Stress Responses

Pain/Stress Response	Relaxation Response
Controlled by the sympathetic nervous system	Controlled by the parasympathetic nervous system
Triggered by pain and stress	Triggered by diaphragmatic breathing (slowing and deepening your breath)
Turned off by diaphragmatic breathing	Reduces pain/stress responses

deep), your muscles also become relaxed. The other problem with shallow breathing is that it keeps your mind tense, too. Your thoughts are more likely to be unsettled, and you are more likely to have trouble calming your thoughts and settling into sleep.

Notice how your breathing changes in the moment before you drop off to sleep. You will find that your breath becomes slow and deep and that your muscles relax completely. While sleeping you are breathing diaphragmatically, and this is part of the restorative aspect of sleep. The goal is for you to experience more diaphragmatic breathing while you are awake: it will help you remain in a state of relaxation, and this will reduce your stress and pain.

Deep Breathing Is Nothing New—Tell Me Something I Don't Know!

The benefits of deep breathing—diaphragmatic breathing—have been described for centuries in Eastern spiritual practices, such as Buddhist meditation. Meditation, a technique used to alleviate both mental and physical suffering, involves diaphragmatic breathing; and just as the breath can provide the gateway to a relaxation response, the breath can serve as the gateway to a meditative state.

Research has shown that long-term meditators have higher levels of resting baseline gamma-band activity in their brains and that they are able to self-induce even greater high-amplitude gamma synchrony during meditation.[114] This information is relevant to pain in three important ways. First, gamma synchrony is thought to play a role in the organization of thoughts and emotions, and may induce synaptic changes in the brain.[115] It is believed that meditation improves a person's ability to regulate thoughts and emotions, and that this regulation extends beyond the time spent meditating and leads to lasting changes manifested in overall greater control. Improved control over thoughts and emotions is critical to pain control, and is covered in more detail in chapter 7.* Second, greater levels of gamma-band activity are associated with increased cortical density and improved processing, integration, and transfer of information between the hemi spheres of the brain;[116] again, suggestive of improved learning. Third, meditation and diaphragmatic breathing involve a highly relaxed state, one that is linked to increased action of the neurotransmitter GABA.† GABA, it turns out, acts to calm the nervous system. It is also linked to changes in the brain, known as neuroplasticity (neuro = brain cell, plastic = changeable).[117] Neuroplasticity is the changing of the brain and the forming of new neural networks. This is an important concept because the goal is to train your mind and body toward the relaxation response and away from the automatic stress and pain responses. You are forming new thought and behavior patterns—all of which encode and change your brain.

Diaphragmatic breathing and meditation are two pathways to help you harness the power of your brain for pain control. Given this, it is

---

*Cortical density is an index of neuronal density in the cortical region of the brain.

†Wikipedia: "Gamma aminobutyric acid (GABA) is the chief inhibitory neurotransmitter in the mammalian central nervous system. It plays a role in regulating neuronal excitability throughout the nervous system. In humans, GABA is also directly responsible for the regulation of muscle tone."

no mystery why pain psychologists often teach clients about diaphragmatic breathing in the first few sessions of treatment. Diaphragmatic breathing is a valuable technique that helps you manage pain because it diverts you from two main pitfalls of pain: (1) focusing on the pain and thus unwittingly worsening the pain; and (2) having stored pain/stress responses in your body that worsen your pain. Instead, with diaphragmatic breathing your nervous system is calmed; practiced over time, regular calming creates lasting changes in brain and body. You are retraining your mind and body to return to a "pain-free" state.

You may have heard about diaphragmatic breathing at some point. Pregnant women often learn about Lamaze breath technique in childbirth classes, and this is one form of diaphragmatic breathing. Singers often learn about diaphragmatic breathing in voice classes, and others may have learned about it in a yoga class. The technique I am describing here is not necessarily different from those other techniques. What is different is that **most people with chronic pain do not use these techniques regularly enough to change their experience of chronic pain**. Think of these techniques as medicine. It's not enough to take a medicine once every week or two. If your doctor prescribes a medicine, chances are you take it regularly, probably several times per day to make sure you always have a therapeutic dose of medicine in your blood. Relaxation skills are powerful mind-body medicine that should be dosed regularly to derive their full benefit. Every time you practice the techniques remind yourself that you are dosing your medicine, countering the effects of pain, and training your nervous system away from pain. So if you have heard of these skills before but are not using them now, it will be important to dust them off and begin using them regularly.

A common mistake people make is to only use the skills in times of bad pain—almost as a Band-Aid—to help get them through a pain crisis. Certainly, using these coping skills can help with severe pain. But if you use the skills daily and regularly, you will do more than just help yourself get through bad moments—you will actually be treating the lasting consequences of chronic pain you have been living with. Be sure to practice these skills when you are not in severe pain and are feeling relatively comfortable because you will achieve deeper states of relaxation when you start out with less stress/pain, and therefore can better train your brain and body because there is less resistance.

While the goal is to create lasting changes in the brain and body—and this takes time—you will be surprised what a difference the relaxation makes in your pain and in your sense of calm in the present moment.

Breath Awareness

Take a moment now to focus on your breath. What do you notice? Is your breath short and shallow or deep and elongated? Are you able to notice whether you breathe high up in your chest, or whether you bring each breath down into your body, so that your lower belly is engaged with each breath? Bring awareness to your breath and observe the following characteristics of your breath:

- Notice the size of your breaths. Do you take big, deep breaths or small breaths?
- Notice the rate of your breath. Is your breath slow, quick, or somewhere in between?
- How many breaths do you average per minute?
- Are you a "chest-only" breather or a diaphragmatic breather?
- Recall how your breathing changes when you are in severe pain. Do you tend to hold your breath? If so, when?

Take in one very large breath now. Hold it briefly, then very slowly exhale completely.

Beth's Tips for Breath Work

Be gentle with yourself. It may take time to feel like you've "got it." Just start where you are and give your breath work a bit of attention each day. Remember that it took years for your old breathing patterns

Steps for Breathing into the Relaxation Response (Diaphragmatic Breathing)

1. Find a quiet place and make yourself as comfortable as possible (seated or lying down).

2. Bring your awareness to your breath. Closing your eyes will help you tune your attention to your body.

3. Notice whether your breath is tight or nice and relaxed.

4. Place one hand on your abdomen (just below your belly button).

5. Now focus on slowing down your breath.

6. As you slow your breath, your breath naturally deepens. This is good!

7. Imagine that you are slowly drawing each deep breath all the way down to your abdomen. You may place the palm of one of your hands below your belly button. As you breathe deeply, imagine that you are breathing into the palm of your hand.

8. Allow your abdomen to expand slightly with each breath, so that your hand is able to feel the gentle rising and falling of your abdomen as you breathe. This gentle rising and falling in your abdomen signals that you are engaging your diaphragm—you are now breathing diaphragmatically.

9. Allow yourself to notice the feelings of relaxation spreading throughout your body as your breath continues to expand in your abdomen.

10. Allow yourself to sink deeply into the rhythm of your breath and to be soothed by it.

11. If you notice your mind thinking or wandering, gently bring your awareness back to your breath, back to breathing slowly and deeply.

12. You may notice your hands and feet become warmer as your blood vessels open. You may feel muscle tension begin to melt away. Allow yourself time to enjoy this experience.

to be established, so it may take some practice to shift them. Don't be discouraged by any initial roadblocks; almost everyone hits them. Have patience with yourself and focus on enjoying the mini breathing vacations. Leave your cares behind you for a moment while your sole focus becomes relaxing your breath. Know and trust that if you practice regularly, good results will come.

Practice breathing diaphragmatically several times per day. Do this for 5–10 minutes at a time. *The more you practice the easier it gets.* Remember that you are retraining your mind and body. The body and the brain learn best through consistent, frequent practice. Think about an athlete who prepares their mind and body for competition: they train every day. Or think about a mental athlete preparing for a memory test: they also train every day. The brain changes through repetition. With daily practice the relaxation response soon will be second nature to you!

Begin the easy way. The easiest way to learn to breathe diaphragmatically is to practice when you feel relatively calm and are not in a pain crisis. Over time you will develop confidence and good skill, and then you can begin applying your skills in more challenging situations when pain is high. Eventually, you will find that you can go on autopilot and more easily trigger your relaxation response even in the midst of a pain or stress crisis.

A guided audio CD can work wonders. Use the CD that accompanies this book. Many other standard relaxation audio CDs are also commercially available. Find one that works for you and use it regularly. Brenda's story (which follows) illustrates the difference to be gained by regular use.

To fully treat chronic pain, consider the relaxation response as medicine that you dose several times daily. Regular doses of relaxation medicine will allow you to achieve a continuous state of calm. While even occasional doses of the relaxation response are beneficial, with regular dosing you will experience its full and powerful impact on your nervous system. Brenda is one patient I treated whose life was transformed by frequent use of the relaxation response.

༂ ༄

Brenda's Story

Brenda is a 40-year-old woman who attended my pain class. Complications from a neck surgery she had 6 months before had left her with neuropathic pain that extended down both legs. Bad reactions to a prescribed medication also left her with tremors and an unsteady gait. She was forced to give up her job as a private detective—a job she loved. Her average pain level was 6 out of 10, but her pain would regularly spike when she was stressed or when she pushed herself hard. In the class she learned diaphragmatic breathing and I guided everyone through a 20-minute muscular relaxation session. Afterward, participants talked about their experiences.

Brenda was surprised at her results. "What I notice is that I hold my breath," she said. "I don't breathe right, and I'm not sure that I ever have. I know for certain that as long as I've had my severe pain, I have been holding my breath." She described how she shifted her breath by inhaling deeply until her lower abdomen expanded slightly.

Brenda practiced diaphragmatic breathing daily. I gave her a guided relaxation audio CD (similar to the one that accompanies this book) that includes diaphragmatic breathing and muscle relaxation, and she began using it twice daily. I saw her back in clinic a week later, and she was happy that she was getting results. I asked her what she was noticing as she practiced with the CD. "My muscles relax, and I just feel peaceful and at ease. I literally feel the tension leave my body. I cannot believe what a difference this makes."

Brenda continued to use the breath work over the weeks and found that she was able to release physical and mental tension on a regular basis. She became good at using the relaxation response. Essentially, she learned how to engage her parasympathetic nervous system—the part of the nervous system that modulates stress and pain. By practicing regularly, *she was shaping her own nervous system toward health and well-being*.

Brenda regularly monitored her breath and adjusted it when she found her breathing was short or "tight." Regular use of relaxation response did not eliminate Brenda's need for opioids, but she found that she took less of them and she was able to stop at least one of her other medications. Most importantly, she was thrilled that she achieved these results on her own—through her own work. She had missed the sense of accomplishment she had derived from being a great investigator. Now she was channeling her desire for achievement toward herself and her pain management goals, and she was pleased with her results. At our last session she was excited to report she was returning to part-time work

❧   ❧

The Power of Advanced Relaxation Technology

Recently, health researchers and neuroscientists have unveiled clues about how the age-old techniques of diaphragmatic breathing and the relaxation response can be improved upon. You can use advanced technology to create an enhanced relaxation response—one that allows for deeper encoding and quicker results.

❧   ❧

Debbie's Story

At age 50, Debbie had been living with chronic pain for 15 years. While she had tried psychological counseling and all types of pain medicine, nothing seemed to help her pain. One connection she had observed was the strong tie between her stress and her pain. She had strained, stressful relations at home and at her job, and she was miserable with her pain and feeling out of control. She was at her wits' end when I met her in clinic.

My first step with Debbie was teaching her how to use the relaxation response (diaphragmatic breathing and guided muscle relaxation). She began using this twice daily, and a week later she reported some improvement in her stress and her pain. She certainly felt calmer.

113

The second step involved combining the standard relaxation she was already using with a brain-changing trick known as *bilateral touch* that allows for more rapid change to take place. Using bilateral touch with relaxation can give you a fast-tracked response that helps your nervous system calm quickly and deeply. I explained the technique to Debbie as follows.

Imagine a line running down your body that exactly divides it in half. The brain is also divided in half, split into hemispheres. Each hemisphere corresponds with the opposite side of your body. Bilateral touch involves quickly touching one side of the body, then quickly touching the other side. In other words, each side of the body is touched—or lightly tapped—quickly and in alternating order to stimulate the hemispheres of the brain. It turns out that stimulating the hemispheres of your brain in rapid, alternating order has powerful effects on your brain, and on your experience of relaxation and pain.

For bilateral touch, it doesn't matter *where* you touch your body—you could touch your feet, your knees, or your arms and gain the same result. I find it easiest to touch the backs of the client's hands or the tops of their knees—but it could be anywhere that is not sensitive or painful. Debbie chose her knees. While she sat with her eyes closed, I lightly tapped on her knees for between 5 and 10 minutes as I guided her to breathe diaphragmatically and release tension from her body.

Debbie had an immediate transformation. She could not remember feeling so calm and peaceful. She then went home and twice daily self-treated by listening to her standard relaxation audio CD while using the bilateral touch method I taught her. Sometimes she tapped on her knees, sometimes her arms. When she chose her knees, she placed one hand on each knee and tapped lightly with her index fingers in rapid, alternating order. When she chose her arms, she would cross her arms and tap on each upper arm with her index fingers.

Debbie returned after using bilateral touch and relaxation for a week and reported a dramatic change. Work was easier. While she had previously avoided her coworkers and kept to herself, she found herself interacting with people joyfully—something that was foreign to her. Her anxiety was diminished, and she felt connected to a positive expectation for the new work year. She was ruminating less and generally *felt* better. She had tears in her eyes as she described the difference she was experiencing. She was partially in disbelief, and yet grateful for her undeniable result. We celebrated her success together.

Six weeks later her results were maintained. She had newfound confidence, a strong ability to be clear with herself and others, and her best pain control in 15 years. She still had pain to manage, but she felt in control.

ᔥ• •ᔦ

To be sure, not everyone will experience Debbie's dramatic improvement. Regardless, I can say that over the past 7 years of using the technique with patients, I have observed that bilateral touch and binaural sound deepen and strengthen the relaxation response and enhance pain relief.

What Is Binaural Sound?

Binaural sound* works on the same principle as bilateral touch: each hemisphere of the brain is being stimulated quickly and in alternating order. Binaural sound involves rapid tones or beats being heard in one ear, then the other, in repeating, alternating order—a sonic "tapping." Binaural sound is best experienced with headphones. It has the same calming effect as bilateral touch, and later I discuss how bilateral stimulation can be experienced visually.

---

*The science of binaural sound dates back to 1839 when German experimenter Heinrich Wilhelm Dove discovered that binaural sound had a powerful effect on the brain. Many years later, in 1973, Gerard Oster published "Auditory beats in the brain" in *Scientific American*. Oster described how binaural beats essentially entrain the brainwaves, making the brain more programmable.

Binaural Sound Decreases Fentanyl Use

In 1999 binaural sound was first studied for pain control during surgery.[119] The study aimed to test whether patients who listened to an audiotape with binaural sound during surgery would require less anesthesia than patients who listened to tapes of relaxing music or tapes with no sound (placebo).

All of the patients in the study were given an opioid medication, fentanyl, through an IV catheter. In the surgical setting, the purpose of the fentanyl is anesthesia, and it also serves to stabilize blood pressure and heart rate—two indicators of pain and stress. The patients were under anesthesia when the various tapes and sounds were played, so they were "blind" as to which study group they were in. The researchers discovered that the patients who listened to the binaural sound needed much less IV fentanyl to maintain their heart rate and blood pressure compared to patients who listened to the classical music or the blank tape!

In 2004 different scientists replicated these findings in bariatric surgery patients. Patients who listened to binaural sound during surgery required less anesthesia than patients who listened to a blank audiotape.[120] Collectively the surgical studies tell us that binaural sound acts at the unconscious level to help stabilize heart rate and respiratory rate, two markers of stress, pain, and nervous system arousal.

Binaural Sound in Chronic Pain

Binaural sound appears to act at the unconscious level to help reduce markers of stress and pain, and it reduces the need for anesthesia. Although we don't yet know how or why it works, the research hints that binaural sound has a calming effect on the human nervous system. Now we are applying this advanced technology to chronic pain. At Stanford University in 2013, I developed the audiofile/CD that accompanies this book, "Enhanced Pain Management: Binaural Relaxation." During the 20-minute guided relaxation exercise, I narrate listeners through diaphragmatic breathing and progressive relaxation designed specifically for people with chronic pain. Layered behind my voice are subtle binaural sounds that serve to enhance the brain's relaxation response. I created the binaural audio CD to capitalize on the fact that binaural sound and standard relaxation techniques calm the nervous system. *Combining* binaural sound with the relaxation response may prove particularly potent for reducing pain and suffering.* The binaural audiofile can be a particularly useful tool for people who have great difficulty with meditating or sitting still because the listener is directed to focus on something—the mind gets to stay busy in a helpful way.

What Is EMDR?

Eye movement desensitization and reprocessing therapy (EMDR) is the most common treatment that uses bilateral visual stimulation. EMDR, developed by Dr. Francine Shapiro, was first tested as a treatment for psychological trauma, and it has since been applied to other medical symptoms. A trained EMDR therapist uses a specific treatment protocol with clients. Classically, the treatment involves having the client move their eyes from side to side. The therapist may hold their hand in front of the client's face and move their finger from side to side; the client holds their head still while they follow the therapist's finger movement with their eyes. The client's eye movements resemble what occurs during the rapid eye movement (REM) stage of sleep. In addition to eye movements, EMDR may also use other forms of bilateral stimulation, such as binaural sound or bilateral touch. In other words, EMDR uses the methods described by Oster and used in the surgical experiments, and those methods are paired with a protocol used by trained therapists.

EMDR is effective treatment for post-traumatic stress disorder (PTSD). People diagnosed with PTSD have experienced some sort of trauma, such as physical or sexual abuse or war-related combat. A

---

*At Stanford we are conducting studies to determine the additive value of binaural relaxation for chronic pain compared to standard relaxation therapy.

person can also be traumatized by believing that they, a loved one, or another person are in grave danger. PTSD is a moment of trauma or shock that encodes deeply in the nervous system and remains "stuck" as a continuous and extreme stress response. Some other common symptoms of PTSD include experiencing flashbacks where one feels as though they are reliving or reexperiencing the trauma. Flashbacks feel like real experiences—not just memories—and during a flashback a person may behave as if they are back in the moment of the trauma. The brain and the body believe and respond as if they are continually under siege.

EMDR has been shown to be a more effective treatment for PTSD than standard care or a pill placebo, and has shown better longevity of treatment effects than fluoxetine, a commonly prescribed antidepressant better known as Prozac. PTSD is resolved in roughly 85 percent of people who receive the treatment. By pairing bilateral touch, binaural sound, or bilateral visual stimulation with therapist-guided psychological techniques, the brain may begin to understand that there is no current threat and that the red alert may be stopped. This then leads to normalization of stress responses, thought patterns, and the resolution of flashbacks and other symptoms. In other words, the nervous system is finally calmed, and this calm state is *encoded* and becomes permanent. Collectively, the EMDR studies provide specific information to show that bilateral stimulation can calm the nervous system to reduce the lasting effects of psychological trauma.

PTSD and pain are similar in that they both trigger the danger alarm in the brain. While you may not have PTSD, the binaural CD and audiofile that accompanies this book will allow you to better train your nervous system to a calm state, thereby dampening any "danger alarms" that accompany pain and anxiety. Another study found that rapid bilateral eye movements create changes in how the two hemispheres of the brain communicate with each other. Another study found that the eye movements increased processing *within* each hemisphere of the brain.[121] Increased communication within the brain allows for the laying down of new pathways in the brain, a marker of encoding or learning.

Shift Your Thoughts and Emotions to Reduce Your Need for Prescription Opioids

Let nothing dim the light that shines from within.

—Maya Angelou

As the Brain Goes, So the Pain Goes

You know that your pain is not "all in your head," yet your mind has a powerful influence on your experience of pain. How you *think* about your pain—and the meaning you give to your pain—will make your pain better or worse.

In this sense, your mind is like the volume dial on a radio. The sound of the radio broadcast represents your pain condition—maybe a failed surgery, migraines, or a disease. The volume dial—your mind—controls how softly or loudly you experience your pain. You can use the power of your mind to turn the dial down and have less pain; it won't take away your entire pain condition, but it can give you back a critical level of control over your pain. And in the context of this book, this outcome usually means fewer pills.

Let's take a step back from pain and think about the impact and influence of emotions on how you approach living.

You are well aware that your thoughts, beliefs, and emotions influence your life. If you miss a flight, your first thought might be "this is horrible!" followed by a feeling of panic. In the next moment, your thought process might shift: "I didn't plan for this, but it looks like I have an extra day here. I will need to make a few phone calls back home." After that, you might think that this missed flight is a great opportunity to do something positive (relax, visit a museum, etc).

In this example, the shift in your thought process changed your experience from one of panic and dread to one of acceptance and excitement about the day ahead. Similarly, with pain, your thoughts have the power to change your experience of your body, your pain, and your life. The same is true for your beliefs and emotions.

Consider that your mind is so powerful it can determine whether a pain treatment will work or not! It is commonly thought that the most important medical treatments involve surgery, doctor visits, or pharmaceuticals. Some evidence hints that the mind may very well be the most important factor in pain treatment.

A research group from the United Kingdom led by Dr. Irene Tracey conducted an experiment that produced fascinating results showing the power of the mind, expectations, and beliefs.[122] The researchers studied 22 healthy volunteers in a pain experiment. The participants were placed in functional magnetic resonance imaging (fMRI) scanners so their brain patterns could be tracked while they were exposed to a painful heat stimulus on their legs. The average initial pain rating for the study group was 66 (0–100 scale).

Each participant rated their pain level and had an IV catheter placed in one arm. Participants were unaware that they were receiving a strong opioid through their IV lines. The researchers wanted to know how well the opioid would work when the participants did not know about it and were not expecting it. The average initial pain rating of 66 dropped to 55 after the opioid was introduced—not much reduction in pain! The opioid dose was kept constant.

Next, the researchers *told* the participants that they would begin receiving an opioid painkiller through their IV line. Once the participants began *expecting* the pain medication, their pain ratings dropped to 39! Keep in mind that the opioid dose remained constant and had been introduced well before this time.

The dose was kept constant as the researchers next told participants that the painkiller would be stopped—but in reality it was *not* stopped. Based on the belief that they were receiving no opioid medication, participants reported having more pain, and their pain ratings increased to 64—very close to their average baseline pain rating of 66. The researchers correlated the participants' pain scores with their fMRI scans. The brain scan images showed increased blood flow in regions of the brain associated with pain processing and thus corroborated the participants' report of increased pain—**pain generated purely from the belief that they were not receiving any opioid medication**. This experiment showed that beliefs and expectations influence their pain intensity and determine how well treatment works. In this study, beliefs and expectations were more powerful than the opioids. What this means in everyday life is that if you expect pain, you will get pain—*even when taking opioids.*

This small but important study gives clues for how you can harness the power of your mind to change your pain—*really*. You already know that the pain signals in your body are registered and interpreted by your brain, and your brain is your "pain center." Brain imaging studies show that patterns of brain regions activate or "turn on" when a person is in pain.[123,124] Focusing on your pain and how terrible it is also lights up these pain regions in your brain.[125,126] In other words, **just by focusing on pain and anticipating pain,**[127] **you can literally grow pain in your brain and thus grow your pain experience in your body**. And as it turns out, these areas of the brain are most closely linked to emotions of suffering—fear, worry, and sadness. These same emotions not only enhance pain but also diminish the effect of pain treatment.[128]

If you expect your pain to worsen, it will.

Your expectations influence what you feel—emotionally and physically—and therefore your pain. For better or for worse, your thoughts and your emotions change your experience of pain. Negative thoughts and emotions lead to more and worse pain by amplifying pain processing in your central nervous system.

Pain catastrophizing (ka-TAZ-tro-fi-zing)[129] is a negative cascade of distressing thoughts and emotions about actual or anticipated pain. It is when a person remains focused on their pain, magnifies it with their thoughts, is unable to think of anything but their pain, and feels helpless about it. Pain catastrophizing is not black or white—it is a continuum of thinking and feeling. It is natural for everyone to struggle from time to time, but it is important to understand catastrophizing and how to stop it because it is toxic for pain. If you recall my story in Chapter 1, I was clearly catastrophizing my pain, and without knowing it I was making things worse for myself.

Almost 30 years of research has shown the negative effects catastrophizing has on pain, health, and well-being. Across all different kinds of pain conditions, catastrophizing is one of the most important factors—it determines whether some people get well or sick, how quickly people recover from surgery, and whether pain treatments work. Catastrophizing shows us the incredible power our thoughts and feelings have on our bodies and on our health.

Here are some facts about pain catastrophizing:

+ Catastrophizing leads to greater pain intensity.[130–132]

+ People who catastrophize have poorer outcomes after surgery.[132,133] Catastrophizers stay longer in the hospital and have greater pain after surgery, and their pain is more likely to become chronic. Thus, following surgery, catastrophizers may need more pain medication for longer periods of time.

* Catastrophizers are more likely to be depressed—but these are two different things. You can be a catastrophizer without being depressed.[134]

* Catastrophizers have a poorer response to multidisciplinary pain treatment.[135,136]

* Catastrophizing can be more important for pain outcomes than the characteristics of your disease or pain condition.[137]

* Catastrophizers are more likely to *develop* chronic pain after surgery or from an acute injury.[138,139]

* People who catastrophize have a *reduced response to opioids,*[21] just like the people in the experiment who thought they were not getting IV opioids.

Focusing negatively on your pain strengthens the pain signaling in your brain.[140,141] Furthermore, *catastrophizing doesn't just grow pain in the brain; it also keeps it there.*[142,143]

Results from brain imaging research show that emotional processing is overactive in people with chronic pain. These same emotional areas of the brain contribute to the experience of constant pain.[144–148] Catastrophizers are less able to disengage from and suppress pain. No wonder pain is worse in catastrophizers! A vicious cycle of catastophizing ⟶ pain ⟶ catastrophizing ⟶ pain can easily take root and contribute to the need and use of opioids.

Catastrophizing feeds your chronic pain experience. You can learn to take control. You may lessen your suffering by using skills and tools that control your brain patterns of thought and emotion.

Imagine for a moment that your chronic pain is a small campfire. Focusing on your pain, how bad it feels, and feeling helpless about it is like dousing the campfire with gasoline—it can cause *more* pain. The fire grows larger because, with your negative thoughts and emotions, you are unwittingly lighting up areas of your brain that amplify pain. You become hypervigilant, constantly monitoring your body for pain and focusing on analyzing every sensation to determine whether it is painful. Your fire grows larger.

Rather than pouring gasoline on the fire and unwittingly making your pain worse, you can learn to put the gasoline can down. This means learning how to stop negative thoughts and feelings as quickly as possible. Doing so requires learning how to get yourself to a mental and emotional "neutral" where you are not using the power of your mind against yourself, thus creating distress and more pain.

Take the quiz that follows on pages 126–128 to find out whether you can improve your pain by changing thinking patterns about pain. Information in this chapter will give you the road map to get back on track by using your mind to lessen your pain.

Tom is a patient I worked with in clinic. His story shows how he was using the power of his mind to worsen his pain—and how he learned to turn it around for himself.

✒ ✒

Tom's Story: An example of pain catastrophizing

Tom was awakened at 5 A.M. by a deep aching in his bones. He was tired, he hurt, and he was frustrated. He had an important meeting to attend this morning and he had no time for pain. He tossed and turned for half an hour, desperately trying to catch some precious last moments of sleep. In the meeting he was going to give a sales pitch to an important client and could not afford to be off his game. His pain was severe, and he was growing increasingly worried that his pain would distract him during the meeting. He kept focusing on his pain, monitoring it to see if it was getting worse as he feared it would, and he couldn't stop thinking about how awful it was.

Tom thought that if his pain continued to worsen over the next few hours he might need to cancel the meeting at the last minute—and he knew that both the client and his boss would be annoyed with him at best, angry at worst. Thinking about it now, Tom felt a hard lump in his throat as he swallowed; evidence of his distress and feelings of helplessness over his pain. He imagined the consequences of his pain worsening. "Why should I even bother getting out of bed?" he thought to himself. "If my pain gets any worse I'm bound to make a disastrous mistake today. I'm already tired and foggy-headed and I know it will be downhill from here. I should probably cancel the meeting now."

Tom's catastrophizing was worsening his distress and pain, and it was preventing him from being able to think clearly, problem-solve, and make good decisions about what to do next.[129] You may recognize parts of Tom's story in yourself and how you relate to pain from time to time.

Tom's Treatment for Catastrophizing

Tom learned that the way he was thinking about his pain was only making him more upset and his situation worse. He also found that when he expected his pain to create a disaster in his day it often did. Instead of focusing on everything that was out of his control, he learned to start focusing on small things that he *could* control. The day before important meetings he focused on preparing himself so that his night was freed up for relaxation: a hot bath, his relaxation response CD, and early to sleep.

He began holding a positive expectation for having a good day, but also knew that if he awoke with pain, he would follow a concrete action plan: (1) remain calm; (2) focus on relaxing his breath, mind, and body; and (3) take medication as prescribed. He developed a pain plan with his work supervisor. If his pain was bad, he would call in to the conference. Just having a plan in place reduced Tom's stress, and his ability to call in to meetings meant he started missing less work. And if he was having

continues on page 129

125

Pain Catastrophizing and Pain Stress Quiz*

A. When I'm in pain, I have a hard time focusing on anything else.
    1. Rarely; I can focus my mind on other things.
    2. Occasionally
    3. Often or always; all I can think of is how bad my pain is.

B. I tend to worry that my pain will get worse.
    1. Rarely or never
    2. Sometimes
    3. Often

C. I feel helpless over my pain.
    1. Rarely; there are many things I can do to help my pain (besides just taking medication).
    2. Sometimes
    3. Often

D   When I'm in pain, I'm good at focusing on what I can do to help myself rather than staying stuck in negative thinking.
    1. Most of the time
    2. Sometimes
    3. Almost never; can't see beyond the negative when I'm in pain.

E. I tend to worry about the possibility of pain coming on.
    1. Rarely
    2. Sometimes
    3. I often worry about the possibility of pain coming on.

_____

*This quiz is not diagnostic. It is meant to give you a general understanding of how your thoughts and emotions are influencing your pain. Virtually everyone can benefit from improving the coping skills taught in this chapter.

F. When I feel pain, I tend to keep monitoring how bad it is.

   1. Rarely

   2. Some of the time

   3. Often; I tend to continually monitor my pain, checking to see if it's getting worse.

G. I take medication in advance of pain because I'm keyed up thinking the pain will come on.

   1. Never

   2. Occasionally

   3. Often; if I think I might be feeling pain, I will quickly reach for medication.

H. I regularly use strategies—other than medication—to calm myself down when I'm in pain.

   1. True

   2. Somewhat true; but I know I can learn more.

   3. False; I do not regularly use strategies to calm myself and lessen my pain.

I. I feel I have pretty good control over my pain.

   1. True

   2. Somewhat true, but I could improve my sense of control.

   3. False; I often feel my pain is out of my control.

J. Even when my pain is severe, I know it will get better.

   1. Almost always

   2. Sometimes

   3. Rarely or never

continues ▶

K. I have adjusted my expectations for myself so I don't feel the pressure to perform as if I didn't have chronic pain.

    1. True; I have changed my goals so they are realistic for me.

    2. Somewhat true, but I could improve here.

    3. False; I still hold myself to my old "prepain" standard and feel like a failure if I fall short.

L. I address any problems assertively in order to keep my stress levels low.

    1. True; I am good at dealing with problems and solving them quickly

    2. Somewhat true.

    3. False; I tend to avoid conflict and stuff my feelings inside of me in order to "keep the peace."

My total score: _____ **Date:** _____

Scoring Key:

12–16: Congratulations, you direct your thoughts in a way that helps your pain—this is what psychologists call positive coping.

17–21: You have some good skills in place but clearly can benefit from learning more about how to use your mind in a way that improves your pain.

22–36: You are experiencing challenges in coping with your pain— you may even be struggling right now. The good news is that you can learn how to cope better. As you continue to read, you will to learn how to work with your thoughts to change your experience of pain and to lessen your suffering. Your ability to control your thoughts and emotions will help you rewire your brain and its responses to pain. If you have trouble applying the knowledge in this book, consider working with a psychologist to help guide you toward positive results.

a really lousy pain day that was helped by nothing, he gave himself permission to cancel work. He learned to talk to himself differently so that he relieved the pressure on himself. He shifted his focus from feeling badly about himself to focusing on taking excellent care of himself when he was in pain. Tom began reminding himself that the sky would not fall at work and that he could regroup the next day when he felt better.

⮕ ⬅

It does not matter whether you have degenerative disk disease, rheumatoid arthritis, or some other medical condition. **Regardless of your type of condition, how you think and feel about your pain (and the other parts of your life) plays a large role in how bad—or good— your pain gets.** You will learn how to regulate your emotions, how to stop catastrophizing, and how to develop positive ways of coping with pain and stress. Then when you catch yourself thinking and feeling negatively, you can steer yourself back to safe ground—before you go down the slippery slope and unwittingly make your pain worse.

Catastrophizing takes any situation and makes it worse. It can trigger the stress response; and as you now know, a stress response will worsen your pain. Bring awareness to your thoughts and how you focus your mind. How you direct your thoughts and your awareness has a very real impact on your body, your pain, your health, your quality of life, and your need for pain medication.

My research and the research of others has offered some initial evidence that catastrophizing causes the body to release inflammatory factors into the bloodstream.[149,150] Inflammation is known to make pain worse, and it can also lead to the worsening of underlying disease or medical conditions. While more research is needed, these studies offer clues about how catastrophizing impacts the body and pain.

Begin to notice yourself catastrophizing—when you focus on the negative and when you feel at the mercy of your pain. Once you catch yourself, it is important to stop catastrophizing as quickly as possible. Over time you will get better at catching yourself catastrophizing and stopping it in the moment.

Five Golden Steps to Stopping and Preventing Catastrophizing

Follow these steps to stop catastrophizing, calm your nervous system, and gain control over your thoughts, emotions and pain.

Step 1. Bring Your Awareness to Your Breath

Catastrophizing begins with your thoughts. For example, you may find yourself worrying about your pain or the situation worsening, or you may focus on how awful it is. You may try to distract yourself and find that your mind goes right back to catastrophizing. The first thing to focus on is calming your nervous system using the skills you've already learned. Then, once your mind and body are calmer, the strategies you use to shift your thinking will be more effective.

To stop catastrophizing, calm your nervous system first; then use strategies to change your thoughts.

As you learned in chapter 6, it is impossible to be in the stress response and the relaxation response at the same time. Catastrophizing triggers a stress response—you have probably felt this yourself, and research also proves this to be true. The antidote is the relaxation response*, and the gateway to the relaxation response is diaphragmatic breathing. Bring your awareness to your breath and begin guiding yourself into diaphragmatic breathing. Allow your breath to calm mind and body as the first step toward stopping catastrophizing right in the moment. Think of diaphragmatic breathing as the "emergency brake" you use when your thoughts automatically begin charging ahead catastrophizing. Focusing your mind on relaxing your breath stops

---

*As stated earlier, catastrophizing is associated with the release of proinflammatory cytokines in the blood. The relaxation response, on the other hand, is associated with anti-inflammatory properties.[157]

catastrophzing because you are no longer focusing negatively on your pain. Simultaneously, relaxing your breath will trigger a relaxation response that will calm your entire nervous system. A calm nervous system is also incompatible with catastrophizing. Mission accomplished!

Step 2: Use Your Self-Soother Action List

Once you have lowered your distress level with a few minutes of calming breathing, the next step is to do something else that is both soothing and distracting. Catastrophizing means you are upset and in need of comfort and support. Giving *yourself* comfort and support in the moment will help you slow and stop the catastrophizing cascade. It doesn't take much. Small actions—like fixing yourself a cup of tea, reading an affirmation, calling a good friend, taking a short walk, journaling, taking a moment to observe beauty, reviewing a short "gratitude" list that you made ahead of time—can go a long way to shifting your energy, changing your thoughts, recalibrating your perspective, and improving your emotions. We cannot physically hug ourselves when we need comfort, but we can essentially "give ourselves a hug" by nurturing ourselves with actions of kindness when we need it most. Recall that part of the definition of cata-strophizing is feeling helpless about pain. Small positive actions serve to stop catastrophizing because they direct you toward things you *can* do to help yourself in the moment. There is hidden power in doing something positive for yourself—even something small!

Create Your Self-Soother Action List in Advance

Your action list will be personal and may look very different than the examples given here. That's OK. Brainstorm about what works for you. Bear in mind that you will problem-solve and brainstorm best when you are relaxed, calm, and comfortable. Make it real by writing your list down on paper or on your mobile electronic device. Keep your handy so you can pull it out quickly the moment you catch yourself catastrophizing. Having your premade list allows you to immediately focus on doing the items on your list without having to problem solve or generate items when you are struggling. Your list will include activities that are soothing and simultaneously serve the purpose of focusing your mind on a positive experience.

Using your soother list will "change the channel" in your brain. At a minimum you are shifting from the pain/stress channel to a neutral channel. Neutral means an absence of stress and emotional charge. Over time, as you practice your mind-body skills and use your soother list often, you will reduce the intensity of catastrophizing and the amount of time you spend catastrophizing. You will stop yourself catastrophizing sooner than you did before. You will catastrophize *less*. You will find that changing the channel in your brain becomes easier over time because you are forming positive pathways in your pain and extinguishing the negative catastrophizing patterns. *You are changing your brain*. You will be able to use your soother list and get to a positive, calm, and nurturing state of mind. This may take some time—so have patience. Focusing on getting your mind to a neutral state is an excellent first goal. When your mind is in a neutral state, you are no longer contributing to your pain and suffering—and this is *fantastic*!

Having one general catastrophizing soother list is a nice place to start. However, I recommend you create several different lists: one for home, one for work, one for when you are with other people, and so on. Each list should include at least five soothing activities that would be fairly easy for you to do in a given situation.

A Sample Soother Action List

Here's an example of a general catastrophizing self-soother action list:

1. Read affirmations.

2. Fix a cup of herbal tea.

3. Review my gratitude list (5–10 things in my life that I feel grateful for).

4. Listen to 5 minutes of the binaural audiofile or a meditation CD.

5. Check back in with breath; diaphragmatic breathing for 5 more minutes if needed.

6. Go for a short walk alone or with a friend.

7. Sit in nature for 10 minutes.

To help stop catastrophizing, it is important to have a list of simple, nurturing things you can do for yourself—it's like giving yourself a hug. It's good self-care. And, pleasure creates interference in your brain's pain circuitry.

Your experiences shape your brain activity, so be sure to expose yourself to the things that will bring you support, comfort, and pleasure.

Create your catastrophizing soother list by jotting down a number of simple and nourishing things you can do for yourself when you are struggling or need restoration. **Create your list when you are not in crisis and keep it in a predictable location.** When you catch yourself catastrophizing or struggling with negativity, pull out your list begin working your way down the list—no need to think or problem-solve. Some days you may only need one soother action to lift you out of negativity. Other days you may need several soothing actions. Go right into *any* behavior that will create a sense of calm nurturing.

My Catastrophizing Soother Action List

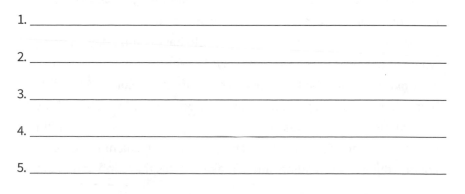

1. _____

2. _____

3. _____

4. _____

5. _____

Focus on being gentle with yourself. Self-compassion is often a foreign concept for people, but it is one of the most important ones, especially if you have chronic pain. When you are having a bad day or a hard time, go through step 1 to help you calm yourself and find center. Now use your self-soother action list and do something nice and nurturing for yourself. It doesn't matter what you choose to do: fix a cup of hot tea, rest for a few moments, call a friend, go outside in the garden, hold your pet, take a warm bath. Your list of nurturing activities will be unique to you—it can be anything that brings you a bit of pleasure and positive focus of your energy in a moment of painful discomfort.

Step 3: Set Realistic Expectations

Having unrealistic expectations is a common pitfall that generates more suffering. You can learn to avoid this trap, and in doing so will give yourself the gift of less pain.

❧ ❦

Matthew's Story

Matthew had a hard time setting expectations that matched his current reality. He had chronic hip and back pain from ankylosing spondylitis, an inflammatory rheumatic condition that causes pain, fatigue, and bone changes. Ankylosing spondylitis can cause the bones in the spine to grow together in some people. Matthew was only 26 years old, but he felt like he had the body of an 80-year-old man. He had to give up a lot of things, including his beloved sports—running and soccer. Some movement and exercise, like walking and swimming, helped his pain. But running and soccer were too jarring and made things worse.

About every week or so Matthew would have a good day—a day when his pain was lower. On these days he would go out and try to run or kick around a ball, to prove to himself that he could. Who could blame him for wanting to have a normal body again? Expecting his body to be like it was before was causing him problems. Repeatedly "testing" his body with activities that flared his pain was causing him problems. For one thing it was leading him to make choices that robbed him of the enjoyment of his "good" days. He might get a few minutes of jogging in, but then he was left with more pain and feelings of disappointment—and this led to him focusing on how bad his pain was and worrying that his pain was never going to get any better.

❧ ☙

Joann's Story

Like Matthew, Joann struggled with her expectations. She was ambitious, and had propelled herself to professional success by pushing herself hard. Despite having migraines, she kept trying to use the same approach that had worked for her all her life: work hard and push through. Now that her migraines were worse, she was no longer calling the shots—her body was; and while it required compromise and adjustment, Joann wasn't prepared to give in or slow down. She kept working long hours with little sleep, and this only triggered more migraines. Once a migraine set in, she was knocked out for at least a day—unable to accomplish anything. She catastrophizes her migraines as soon as they began out of fear of the impact it would have on her work. Once she felt better, she would redouble her efforts to catch up on the work she missed while recovering from the migraine.

Joann was caught in a trap of unrealistic expectations—she was expecting her body to perform as if she didn't have migraines. The problem was she couldn't get away with it any longer. She needed a slower pace and better self-care in order to prevent her migraine episodes. Joann learned to challenge her belief that slowing down would prevent her from meeting her goals. In fact, she found that she was able to accomplish *more* by working at a more reasonable pace because she had fewer down days. Certainly, her overall productivity was lower than it was before she had migraines—she was now working 35 hours each week instead of 50. But given that she now had chronic pain, she found that having realistic expectations allowed her to maximize her productivity and prevent pain flares, and it stopped the catastrophizing.

❧ ☙

Notice whether you have unrealistic expectations that are causing you more distress and suffering. As you know, pain often slows life down considerably. Sure, you may be able to push yourself and work a full day, but at what cost? If you find the cost is more down days, you are probably moving in the wrong direction.

Having expectations that are formed from your past or your peak potential is a setup for stress, pain, and disappointment. Allow your expectations to come into alignment with the body you have *now*, in present time, in this exact moment. In other words, factor in your chronic pain and *also* consider how you are feeling *right now*. In Joann's case, while she set a comfortable 35-hour/week schedule for herself, she still allowed for adjustments each day to accommodate how she was feeling. What seems to be a realistic expectation today may be unrealistic next week if your circumstances or conditions change. If you get lousy sleep one night, you may find that what seemed to be an easy goal now needs revising so you can honor your body's limits as they are, right now. **Become mentally flexible. Allow yourself to adjust your expectations based on how you feel *now*—in present time.**

How to Know If You Have Unrealistic Expectations

Here are a few indicators of having expectations that are not realistic:

- If you find yourself often having pain flares because you push yourself to do more than your body can handle, you probably have unrealistic expectations of yourself.

- If you feel overwhelmed with trying to manage daily life and your pain, you may have unrealistic expectations about what's reasonable for you to manage. Having chronic pain generally means some—or a lot—of your energy is lost to pain. Less energy means less will get accomplished, so this requires an adjustment in expectations.

- If you find yourself caring for other people in your life and neglecting your own self-care, you have unrealistic expectations of yourself.

Come into present time with your body. Just because you could do something easily in the past does not mean it would be wise or healthy for you to do it now. Your chronic pain may have changed your physical abilities. Your body is probably different now, and coming into acceptance about the realities of your physical limitations can go a long way to easing the pressure on yourself.

Beth's Tips

Just because you can doesn't mean you should. Sure, you can do all the yard work in one day or wait on your family hand and foot in one day from dawn to dusk. And then you find yourself knocked out for two days after that, feeling utterly miserable. Don't set yourself up for more pain. Become aware of your choices, your patterns, and how they impact your pain. Pacing yourself and taking frequent breaks will give you time to evaluate how you are feeling and to make realistic adjustments that help you keep your pain low.

Avoid the trap of pushing yourself too hard because you know you can take opioids to mask the extra pain. This is a real trap that will leave you taking more opioids than you should, putting you at risk for more complications and negative side effects. Opioids should not be used to enable you to do things that are not good for you.* If you find yourself doing this often, work with a pain psychologist to help you get out of this bad cycle. Ideally, if taken mindfully, opioids may increase

---

*If you take opioids they should allow you to do more—to function better. Opioids should not be used to allow you to abuse yourself with an unrealistic level of activity.

a person's function—but this is a balancing act. Opioids should not be used to consistently mask the results of bad choices. Freedom from pain and pharmaceuticals is found when you listen to your body and make daily choices that honor your body's limitations.

Honor your body in present time. Honoring your body requires that you set boundaries with yourself and other people to ensure that your body is well cared for. You may have to say no to yourself and to others from time to time because you know that what your body needs is something else: rest, therapeutic exercise, quiet time, sleep, stress reduction. Honoring your body in present time means being willing to shed old, outdated expectations. It also means being willing to shed old, outdated patterns of behavior that no longer serve you.

Those patterns may never have served you well, but with chronic pain you have less capacity and energy to accommodate any patterns that do not serve you positively. Honoring your body in present time means allowing outdated structures to fall away so that you can best care for the body you have now.

Step 4: Be Gentle with Yourself

Be gentle with yourself mentally, emotionally, and physically. Having chronic pain is frustrating, and often people have anger toward their bodies. Some people are aware of their anger; other people may be unaware of how their anger at their body is affecting their life. You may feel angry that your body will not perform the way it used to, and angry that your life is different because your body is different. Without thinking about it, you may almost be saying to yourself: If my body would just cooperate, all of these problems would go away! You may feel betrayed by your body. A sense of deep frustration may bubble to the surface at times. What do you do with those feelings? A common reaction to any anger or frustration is to take it out on the thing or person that is the problem. But in this case, that's you and your body.

Identify and Stop Any Self-Punishment

One of the biggest ways people unwittingly contribute to their own suffering is by punishing themselves for having a body that is limited by chronic pain. They punish themselves by harboring anger at their bodies. They punish themselves by forcing their bodies to do things they know are not good for them—things that probably will bring on more pain. Reflect on yourself for a moment. Can you think of any big or small ways in which you have anger toward your body? Can you identify ways in which your anger or frustration at your body gets channeled into self-punishment? When you feel anger or frustration with yourself, it's a sign that your mind, body, and spirit need a good dose of the opposite: forgiveness, kindness, love, and gentle acceptance. Never underestimate the power of self-forgiveness and self-acceptance in reducing stress and suffering.

Remember, it is human to have anger and frustration. Allow yourself to observe these feelings when they come up, and allow yourself to observe them without judgment. Allow yourself to observe these emotions as you hold kindness toward yourself:

Of course I feel frustrated that I do not feel able to attend the event as I had hoped to. Of course I am disappointed and wish it were different. But right now, I know the best thing I can do is provide excellent care to myself by changing my plans and staying home. I choose to listen to my body, honor its needs, and relax into present time. It may feel as though my body is thwarting me at times, but I know my body is doing its best to serve me well, given all the limitations it has.

In this scenario, the person is choosing to be in the present moment with *what is*, instead of trying to force *what they would like it to be*. So much suffering in life comes from trying to force what one may wish or want. To wish and to want is human. And yet: accepting what *is* empowers you to begin making choices that can improve your pain and your life.

Ironically, I often hear people say, "But if I accept it, it's like I'm giving into the pain. I'm defeated and it wins." Nothing could be further from the truth. **Acceptance of your present-time reality empowers you: it frees you to begin moving forward rather than staying stuck in the past.**

The formula is this: observe your wishes and wants gently, without judgment, and choose to step into what is reality, in present time. You can still have wishes and wants for the future! **The idea is not to give up hopes and dreams and plans. You may wish for the future** *and observe your reality in present time with your current limitations.* It is not an either/or situation; rather, it is both/and. Choose to honor and live from the space of what is so—right now.

ॐ ॐ

Matthew's Story (continued)

Recall that Matthew was having a hard time accepting the fact that he no longer had a "normal" 26-year-old body and that he could no longer run or play soccer. His treatment involved focusing on what he was able to do—given his pain and medical condition—and not on the things he was giving up. He missed the social aspects of running with a group and playing soccer. He felt isolated with swimming and walking alone. He developed a plan to join a walking group and recreational swim club. He especially liked the swim club idea because it offered him the option of participating in local competitions, something he also missed. Matthew learned that he could work with his body and develop a creative compromise that allowed him to still have experiences that brought him joy and enhanced his life.

ॐ ॐ

What you stand to gain from being gentle with yourself:

- A sense of nurturing when you need it most
- A sense of inner peace and relaxation

- Reduced stress

- Alignment between your needs and your choices

- Less pain

- Less need for pain medication

Beth's Tips for Being Gentle with Yourself

Recognize that you are doing your best. In every moment—even those moments when you may slip into catastrophizing or anger—you are simply doing your best in that challenging moment. Avoid reacting and beating yourself up mentally. Allow the slipups to be OK. Observe the situation with curiosity, see if you can learn anything from it, and quickly move on to what you can do to soften within yourself. Even in the face of a slip-up you can claim a victory if you find softness for yourself.

Step outside of yourself. What if your best friend was experiencing the same challenging situation you are facing? What kind words would you offer your dear friend? You may observe yourself giving supportive advice to your friend while being much harder on yourself. While it is a human tendency to be harder on yourself than on others, shifting this pattern will help you cultivate compassion in your life. *Practice talking to yourself as you would speak to your best friend.* It may feel strange, but try it anyway. Any feelings of strangeness are just a sign that you are absolutely on the right track and need to be doing this. Begin allowing yourself the same compassion as you would a loved one struggling with a similar situation. In this sense, you learn to become your own nurturing best friend. You will begin to observe that you are making kinder choices for yourself.

Focus on self-care. Being gentle with yourself means taking good care of yourself in *all ways*. Are you giving yourself enough time to rest? How is your nutrition? Are you exercising regularly according to your medical plan? How is your balance between social and alone time? Is there something in your life that is missing or needs attention? It may sound simplistic, but much of being gentle with yourself involves all the little daily choices you make.

These daily choices—or "behaviors"—make up your daily life and reveal the relationship you have with yourself. Shifting your daily choices so they come into alignment with the goal of taking excellent care of yourself will create a powerful foundation to support your coming into wellness, reduced pain, and reduced stress. **Each and every choice you make has the ability to move you in the direction of better self-care.** Remember that self-care means making choices that consider how you feel *in present time*.

Become comfortable with saying, "I would like to do that, but I am not able to right now." You will certainly find it helpful to say this statement in different circumstances from time to time, whether you are speaking to coworkers, family, friends, or others. In speaking to yourself, you may say, "I would like to do that, but I *choose* not to right now" (as you know, using the language of choice is empowering). Setting limits with yourself and others is a big part of being gentle with yourself. Using this type of language allows you to gently create a boundary. If others push back against your boundary, it can be helpful to know that they are just doing *their* best in their own challenging situation or in their own limited view. Observe their actions with compassion while still holding firm to your original boundary. Repeat your original boundary statement as needed.

≈ ≈

Meredith's Story

Consider the example of Meredith. Meredith has migraines that are made worse by emotional stress, lack of sleep, and overwork. The family holiday dinner party is hosted in Meredith's home each year, and she does the lion's share of the cooking and hosting duties. It is a tremendous amount of work, and although it is physically taxing, in years past she has enjoyed the fact that the family raves about her party and everyone seems to have a good time.

This year, as she sat in my office, she talked about dreading the party. To begin with, she has been having almost daily migraines. Her best friend, Connie, had surgery and Meredith was spending her free time helping Connie with her recovery. Meredith was exhausted and overwhelmed. The holiday party sounded like a huge chore this year.

"Seriously? Just thinking about it and talking about it is giving me a headache," she said. "I don't want to do it, but I feel trapped. Everyone expects it, and I think my sister may have already bought her plane ticket."

Indeed, it was a bit of a trap. If she hosted the party she would suffer for it; if she canceled the party, her family would suffer. The holiday would not be the same.

"Meredith," I said. "If your family knew that hosting the party was causing you to suffer physical pain and emotional stress, do you really think they would want you to do it?" She paused and looked down. "No. I don't think so."

❧ ❦

Meredith's stress was caused by the thought of canceling the party and disappointing the family. Her stress lessened when she decided to use an incredibly powerful tool: honesty. By bringing honesty into the conversation, Meredith was giving her family the opportunity to be supportive of her limitations—or not; however others responded, Meredith was owning her truth. After a little bit of coaching, she was ready to say what she needed to say.

When I saw her next, Meredith was delighted to share with me how it all unfolded.

≈ ≈

"I sent a mass email to the whole family. I let everyone know that I enjoyed hosting the holiday dinner party for the past several years, and that while I had intended to do so again this year, things hadn't gone as planned. I was dealing with an ill friend and with my own chronic pain. As much as I love hosting the party, I knew that doing so wouldn't allow me to take care of myself like I needed. I told everyone that I was deeply disappointed and that I was canceling this year's event at my house." For Meredith, this was a triumph.

"I won't lie; it was hard," she said. "And I think the hardest part was that I wanted to hide the fact that I had pain and couldn't pull it off. Or that I was choosing not to pull it off. But then I figured, hey, if my family really cares about me, they will support me in my health care."

It didn't all go perfectly smoothly. She continued to get some flack from one sister who harped to Meredith about how inconvenient it was to make alternate holiday plans. Rather than getting upset about it, Meredith chose to respond calmly and with empathy. "When she brings it up, I just tell her I understand and that I am disappointed, too." She said. "And it's true. But I don't let her disappointment and her words railroad me into doing something that I know would not be good for me."

≈ ≈

Meredith was well on her way to mastering the art of saying, "I would like to do that, but I am not able to right now."

Step 5: Monitor Your Thoughts to Stop and Prevent Catastrophizing

Catastrophizing is an automatic process that becomes a pattern. First, begin to notice your thought patterns. *Identify your triggers.* When are you likely to catastrophize? You may be more likely when you are exhausted or your other needs are not being met. Or you may find you catastrophize more in other situations, such as when other people are involved or when you feel alone. Take a moment to think about whether you have catastrophized recently. If you can identify a catastrophizing episode, consider the circumstances that were happening at that time. Was there a particular trigger? Do you have other catastrophizing triggers? Gaining an understanding of your catastrophizing triggers will help you better prepare to handle your thoughts and feelings in those circumstances. As a result, you will not be caught off guard as much, you will feel rooted in a plan of action, and you can then quickly begin using your plan to stabilize yourself.

Make it a new habit to tune into your thought content. Tune in several times a day and begin monitoring your thinking. Do you notice any catastrophizing? Could you be gentler with yourself? Are you neglecting opportunities to release stress? Tune into your breath and adjust your breath as needed to expand relaxation in your mind and body. Monitoring your mind and your body throughout the day— just like this—will help you discover opportunities to become gentler and more relaxed. This, in turn, will help keep catastrophizing at bay.

If you find yourself continuing to struggle with catastrophizing after working through this plan on your own, consider working with a pain psychologist or skilled therapist* who can help guide you through your personal roadblocks. You may only need a few sessions with a skilled therapist to jump-start you on your way to mastering your mind-body connection.

Summary

Below is a summary of key points about pain catastrophizing—and how to reclaim your power.

+ Catastrophizing is an exquisite example of the mind-body connection being used to your disadvantage. You can harness the power of your mind-body connection, shape your brain,

---

*For treating catastrophizing it is generally best to choose a therapist who has a strong training background in Cognitive Behavioral Therapy (CBT).

and change your pain experience. You can learn to control your thoughts to improve your pain and overall health.

• Catastrophizing your pain (or other things in your life) can stimulate pathways in your brain that generate more pain.

• Catastrophizing is destabilizing and leaves you more likely to make choices that make pain worse.

• Catastrophizing begins with your thoughts. The quickest way to **stop** catastrophizing is to bring your focus to your breath. and to expand your focus there. Expanding your focus on your breath will take you away from negative thinking and will begin a relaxation response—an antidote to catastrophizing!

• **To best prevent** catastrophizing:
  ▪ Use the binaural audiofile or CD that accompanies this book several times daily.
  ▪ Monitor your thoughts often and treat negativity in its early stages (use your catastrophizing thought stopping action plan!).
  ▪ Set realistic expectations that are rooted in *present time* and account for your current pain and limitations.
  ▪ Above all: **Be gentle with yourself**.

Beyond Catastrophizing: The Power of Your Thoughts

In the "Five Golden Steps" outlined in the preceding section, I talked about the importance of monitoring your thoughts (step 5). This section expands on the importance of your thoughts in gaining control over your pain and suffering.

Our emotions are born from our thoughts. For example, if you hear that a person lost their job you may think, "that's terrible!" You may feel sad for the person and imagine that losing their job is difficult and may create problems for them. Your interpretation of the situation leads to your emotional experience of sadness or sympathy. Now suppose the person who lost their job began painting and started a successful art business that was much more fulfilling than the job they lost. Once it's understood that losing their job led to positive changes in their life, you feel happy for them.

In another example, you could learn that an old friend broke up with his partner and feel badly for him. And yet when you speak with your friend, he informs you that the breakup was his choice and has led to great happiness. When you learn this, you may feel relieved and glad for him.

In both cases, the assumption was that the circumstance of loss was negative. Often, knowing the full context of the circumstance changes how you feel about the situations.

We use our thoughts to make assumptions, judgments, or appraisals—and these determine whether our emotions are positive, negative, or neutral. This is also true for pain. It would be unrealistic to try to appraise pain as being something positive in your life. It is not. But **you can become more *neutral* about pain and other experiences in your life.**

Your thoughts are incredibly powerful—they determine how you feel and the behaviors and choices you make. Combined, these factors will determine your experience and your outcome. The following is an example that shows how different ways of thinking and appraising pain lead to very different experiences of pain—and very different outcomes.

The Power of Thought Shifting

Susan and Carla are two patients of mine who approach their pain very differently. You can see in Table 7.1 on page 148 that Susan and Carla have different thoughts and feelings about their pain and how, as a result, their *pain experience* is very different. When Susan is in pain, she feels helpless and fearful; she tends to withdraw and "waits out" her pain. Carla is action oriented: she has a plan in place and

Table 7.1 Susan and Carla: An example of how different ways of thinking lead to different experiences of pain

	Thoughts	Feelings	Action	Outcome
Susan	My pain is only getting worse; it is absolutely awful. I want to crawl in bed and cry and escape the pain.	Anxiety, fear, helplessness	Curled up in bed. Braced against the pain; waited it out.	Pain was bad; even when it improved, I was stressed about the work I'd missed.
Carla	Oh boy, my pain is bad. I'm going to make some calls now to ease the pressure at work. Next I'm going to go through the steps to relax my breath and body, and slow things down so I can assess and problem-solve calmly.	Grounded, becoming centered	Rescheduled meetings to reduce pressure on myself, listened to relaxation response CD. Kept self-talk positive and solution focused. Fixed a cup of tea to comfort myself.	Pain was terrible, but I put a container around the negative thoughts and stayed focused on doing everything I could to nurture and help myself. I felt better because I reminded myself that the pain would pass, and it did. I was back at work the next day.

starts working through the steps. She is gentle with herself and is flexible, thus expecting less of herself when she is having a bad pain day. She is focused on remaining calm mentally and physically so that she can be a good problem solver with work-related issues.

Whereas Susan deals with her pain by being fearful and passive, Carla copes with her pain by being action oriented—she addresses her pain directly, and she does it calmly. Carla still has bad pain days, but she has fewer of them, and they are less severe because she has a positive outlook and knows that *she can control aspects of her pain*. As a result, she does not feel helpless over her pain, or at its mercy. Pain is something she deals with, but she doesn't let it control her.

Carla has good control over her thoughts, her feelings, her actions, and her outcomes. So can you. Doing so will relieve stress, help you remain calmer in the face of pain, and improve your overall experience. You can notice your pain, recognize it, and then immediately begin working on your plan to help yourself manage it better.

Reprogramming Your Thoughts

Like catastrophizing, general negative mental chatter can be stopped with the relaxation response. The relaxation response counteracts the stress response and helps you get centered and grounded. Again, use the binaural audiofile that accompanies this book to deepen your relaxation response. You can bring in visualization with relaxation to encourage positive expectation. Envision yourself functioning and feeling better, and notice how wonderful it feels to imagine yourself functioning better. Pair your visualization with bilateral touch to help anchor the image and the associated positive emotions. All of these techniques will help quash negative thoughts.

Now let's put everything together to develop a plan for how you handle catastrophizing. Even if you do not catastrophize regularly, developing a plan will help you think and feel better when you are in pain. Your action plan will optimize your sense of control over your pain and your experience. Think about a time when you did not cope well with your pain. Use the coping log presented in Figure 7.1 and write out how you were thinking and feeling. Then write out what you did.

Now, either think about a time when you coped well, or *imagine* how you can direct your thoughts and behaviors to help you have a better experience. Write down what that looks like.

You can download copies of the coping log at the following site:

www.bullpub.com/downloads

Consider filling out a new coping log at least once or twice weekly. Use it as a tool to gauge your progress with shaping your thoughts and implementing your planned positive coping steps; then evaluate your outcome. It is important to check in and see if you feel different after a few weeks of working through your plan. Tracking your progress can (1) help motivate you to stick with your positive coping plan and (2) help you develop a sense of control over yourself and your experience (e.g., "Wow, I followed my plan, did it myself, and it made a big difference!").

Evaluating your progress also often helps you identify any trouble spots. Once you recognize the roadblocks, you can begin developing a plan for how to address them and, ultimately, overcome them!

Figure 7.1   Coping log and positive coping plan

COPING LOG

Provide an example of a time you did not cope well.

When did this happen? _____

What was the situation? _____

_____

My thoughts	My feelings	My actions	My outcome

MY COPING PLAN

Now make it positive. List an example of a time you coped well; or, *imagine* yourself coping well in a chosen situation and use the information you've learned to describe the specifics.

Describe the scenario (real or imagined) where you cope well:

_____

_____

My thoughts	My feelings	My actions	My outcome

Change Your Choices to Reduce Your Need for Pain Medication

Don't forget to love yourself
—Søren Kirkegaard

THE FIRST STEP IN REDUCING YOUR PAIN and your need for pain medication is learning how to change how your mind and body respond to stress (the relaxation response; chapter 6). The second step is learning techniques to specifically change your thoughts, stop catastrophizing, and find comfort (chapter 7). This chapter focuses on the third step: learning how your daily choices—the responsibilities you accept and the limits you either set or don't set—can influence your need for opioids. Daily choices offer great promise for improving pain—and yet they are probably the most overlooked part of the equation.

Opioids and Your Daily Choices

One pitfall associated with opioids is that they may allow you to continue making questionable choices. Recall you are constantly *participating* with your pain in different ways—through your responses, thoughts, and emotions. A large part of whether your pain worsens or improves depends on the **choices** you make.

Dawn's story provides a great illustration of how you can use the power of choice to change your pain and your life.

ॐ ॐ

Dawn's Story

Dawn is a teacher, wife, and mother to a 16-year-old son. She also has severe chronic back pain and fibromyalgia. As we sat in my office, she described how she felt her pain was controlling her life. I spent time asking her about the choices she would make during a typical day. I learned that she would wake up in pain, exhausted. She would take her opioid medication as prescribed, first thing in the morning.

As a teacher, she struggled to work the full days required of her job. She was a valued member of the teaching faculty and would go the extra mile and volunteer to run committees and mentor other teachers. While she enjoyed these extracurricular roles and the kudos she garnered, it took a toll on her energy and her pain. Around midday she would take another dose of her prescribed opioids.*

She would arrive home and prepare the evening meal, then clean up afterward. On the weekends she managed the household chores, including the shopping. She had no energy for exercise. Any spare time was spent preparing lessons for the following week. I learned that Dawn was pushing herself through each workday, then pushing herself at home in the evenings, and then pushing herself on the weekends.

I asked her about her sleep, and she acknowledged that she wasn't getting nearly enough. She was tired all the time. Her nerves were raw. "I am just so tired," she said slowly as tears began to stream down her face. "I'm trying so hard to keep up, but with the pain . . ." One of Dawn's goals in coming to see me was to get off her opioids. She missed her mental sharpness. Also, she knew that if something didn't change she would remain on opioids indefinitely—possibly the rest of her life. She wanted off

---

*Dawn always took her opioids as they were prescribed by her physician.

opioids, but she saw no way out of her current prescriptions with all the pain she was having.*

I asked her what time she went to bed. She was staying up late because it was the only alone time she had with her husband, David. David liked to watch TV in bed, and then around 11 P.M. they would fall asleep. Dawn's sleep was fragmented, and she had trouble falling asleep and staying asleep. She often awoke during the night in pain. For this reason she took another dose of opioids at bedtime. She would awaken early the next morning and begin the whole cycle again.

❧   ❧

Dawn's choices revealed that she was doing much to accommodate other people in her life—her family, her students, the committees. Yet she was doing almost nothing to accommodate herself or her pain.

As with most clients, I first focused on Dawn's sleep because sleep has a direct impact on pain management. In fact, **one of the best predictors of pain intensity on any given day is the amount and quality of sleep a person had the night before.** Most people are aware that their pain worsens when they are tired. Being tired or fatigued is a signal that the body is stressed. Rest is needed for the body to come back into balance, known as **homeostasis.** Dawn was choosing to stay up late. For her, the benefit was that she was spending time with her husband. The downside was that she was cheating herself out of much-needed sleep. As a result, she was waking up exhausted and unhappy, and she had less energy available throughout the day. Her pain worsened the more she struggled with fatigue, and she would take extra opioid medication for this breakthrough pain—pain that she would feel despite taking her normal scheduled dose of opioids.

---

*Dawn wanted off her opioids even before she learned that they are not effective treatment for her two pain conditions: low back pain and fibromyalgia.

Was Dawn's pain mysteriously "breaking through" her regular dose of opioids, or was it the result of her choices? This was the question I invited her to consider. Her sleep choices were increasing her pain, and she was taking more pills to manage her pain. The irony is that **studies show that opioids further disrupt sleep.**[40] Like many people, Dawn was caught in the sleep-opioid trap. While opioids seemed to help her fall asleep, they were actually worsening her sleep quality; as she became more fatigued, her pain would worsen, which in turn required more opioids, which deprived her of restful sleep . . . and so the cycle continued (see Figure 8.1).

Dawn agreed to try an experiment and put sleep at the top of her priority list.* She talked with David about her sleep goals, and they agreed to focus on having quality time after dinner but before bedtime. This would allow Dawn to go to sleep between half an hour and two hours earlier than David. In order to accomplish this goal, Dawn needed help with dinner cleanup. She enlisted the help of David and her son, Connor. Naturally, Connor didn't want to, but Dawn did a great job of holding firm to her goal. If the kitchen was not clean at 9 P.M., she went to bed anyway. She let David take on the role of kitchen monitor. Dawn told herself that if there were things left undone, she would handle it in the morning when she was better rested and better able to face the situation. She allowed herself to sleep in the guestroom on nights when David insisted on watching TV in their bedroom and she needed total silence. If David was willing to forego TV, she slept in the master bedroom with him.

---

*Good sleep behaviors are called "sleep hygiene." Sleep hygiene principles describe ways to improve sleep such as keeping a regular sleep schedule, avoiding napping during the day, avoiding too much stimulation late at night, avoiding bright lights in the evening hours before bed, and so forth. Everyone with chronic pain can benefit from reviewing sleep hygiene principles and making needed adjustments. The National Sleep Foundation offers sleep hygiene education: www.sleepfoundation.org/article/ask-the-expert/sleep-hygiene

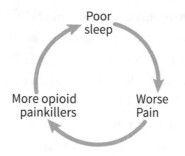

Figure 8.1 The sleep-opioid cycle.

She held fast to her plan and noticed that she felt better in the mornings. She was better able to face the day. Her mood improved because she was not fighting so much fatigue. Her pain improved, and she was able to taper her use of opioids in the afternoons. She was delighted with her progress.

I often see people with chronic pain change their choices and begin to feel better, just like Dawn did. At the moment people feel better, however, they are at risk for making a classic mistake: getting excited about their extra energy and then pushing themselves right back into pain. I encouraged Dawn to avoid this common pitfall and to simply focus on improving her sleep and settling into a life with more energy and less pain. She had worked hard to have less pain, and now she needed to protect it. One thing is certain: **If you look for pain, you will find it.** She noticed that she was always pushing right up against her limit: she was always finding that high edge of pain. She agreed this pattern was not helping her, and she resolved to begin living within a comfort zone instead of a pain zone. Finding her comfort zone required that she make more changes in her daily choices.

Next we took a look at how she was overextending herself at work. Sure, she loved to help others, and she was good at it. But was helping others helpful *to her?* On the positive side, Dawn derived satisfaction and self-esteem from being the go-to person at work, and from being a problem-solving leader at the school. On the downside, giving her time to these other causes meant skipping her lunch hour and staying late after work; this led to an overall stressful feeling of being chronically short on time. It meant she had less personal time and was more tired at home after work and she had more pain from the fatigue and the stress.

Perhaps if Dawn didn't have chronic pain she could handle her work, family, and volunteer demands without ill effects. But given her chronic pain it simply was not possible for her to do all she was doing *and* take excellent care of herself. She was managing to handle work, family, and volunteering responsibilities—but she was doing so *at her own expense*. And she needed the opioid prescription to do it.

Once Dawn understood how her daily choices were maintaining her use of opioids, she resolved to change things in her life and make her health her first priority. She let key people at work know that she needed to reduce her responsibilities for health reasons. She remained on one committee but left her leadership role. She stopped being the go-to person and learned to say no to anything that required giving up her lunchtime or staying later at work than her basic job required. Instead, she started walking 30 minutes each day at lunch, and this was critical: research shows that, **regardless of the cause of low back pain, exercise is one of the best treatments**.[28,151,152] Dawn also had fibromyalgia, and like many other pain conditions, exercise is one of the best treatments for that, too.[153]

The first thing Dawn noticed was that she felt less stressed because others had fewer expectations of her. The second thing she noticed was that she had more free time. She resisted the temptation to fill this time with work and instead used it to focus on her pain and stress management. Determined to reduce her opioid use even further, she practiced the relaxation response at lunch and again right at the end of her teaching day—times when she would have been attending extra meetings.

Within a month she returned to clinic, smiling. "I just feel better," she said. "All-around better. I still have pain, but my pain is not controlling me. I feel in control. Actually, I *am* in control. I feel like I have myself back, but it's even better because for the first time I am focusing on what I need."

Dawn had a big fear of not "being there" for her family or for her work. Part of her identity was wrapped up in being a caretaker. She had an understandable desire to give to others, but she had not thought about what it was costing her. She was surprised to learn that if she scaled back and invested in taking excellent care of herself, she was actually more available to enjoy the time she did spend with her family, students, and coworkers. She was able to spend quality time with David and Connor on the weekends because she was better rested and less stressed. She came to realize that when she felt better, she could actually be more giving. She noticed that the quality of her work improved because she was no longer in a daily state of low-level crisis. In fact, she discovered that setting limits and taking better care of her own needs made her more focused and efficient at work. Even as she was spending less time working, she was getting at least as much done as before.

One technique that helped Dawn was to take an inventory of her choices and to list for each one the benefits of the choice and its impact on her pain (see Table 8.1 on pages 160–161). Once she understood how each choice was affecting her pain, she could make decisions that supported her goals of reduced pain and use of opioids.

Now think about your daily choices: what you get out of them and what they cost you in terms of your pain. Then think about how you can begin choosing differently in order to reduce your "pain cost." Use the template presented in Figure 8.2 on page 162 to document your own benefit/pain cost analysis (the template is also available online at www.bullpub.com/downloads).

Even if you do not write out every single choice you make, begin thinking about *every* choice in terms of how it affects your pain. Each choice has an impact on your pain in one direction or the

Table 8.1   Expense Sheet: Dawn's Choices

CHOICE	BENEFIT (What do I get out of it?)	PAIN COST
Making dinner after work	I get a feeling of satisfaction from caring for my family.	I'm more tired and in more pain in the evening. I don't get a break after work—or all day, for that matter.
Being a committee leader	I get to be the leader; I feel good about helping solve problems and making things better for the kids.	Working extra hours really takes a toll on my energy and my pain. By the end of the day, I am spent.
Staying up late	I enjoy spending time alone with David.	Not sleeping enough makes for a rough next day. I find I need more pain medication.
Working through lunch	This helps me get on top of my workload and in that sense reduces some stress.	Not taking a break at lunch means my pain is worse in the afternoon.
Overworking	I feel good about myself when I am very productive.	My pain is flared and I need more painkillers—then I feel guilty about that because my goal is to take *less* pain medication, not more.
Going to the gym	I feel good about following through with my medical plan.	While I don't always enjoy exercise, my pain improves when I do it regularly.

other. Some choices have a bigger impact than others. Notice which choices you make and observe the **pain cost** of each choice. Then think about whether you are ready to change some of your high "pain cost" choices. Seek to lower the pain cost profile of your choices by making pain management your first priority, which means getting

CHOICE	BENEFIT (What do I get out of it?)	PAIN COST
Doing the laundry	It's easier to do it myself than fighting with Connor about it.	It's one more thing I have to do on my never-ending list, which means less time for me and for stress/pain management. (I'm also spoiling Connor and setting him up for problems with his future spouse!)
Hosting the holiday dinner	The extended family expects me to host it, and I like meeting expectations.	Holidays are an overwork disaster for me when I'm the host. My pain goes through the roof. I do it so I don't feel bad about disappointing others, but I feel physically miserable for it!
Napping on the weekends	I am so tired from the workweek that napping allows me to catch up on my sleep.	Napping throws off my nighttime sleep schedule, so I stay up late on Sunday. I'm usually exhausted on Monday morning—and have more pain.
Choosing not to confront Connor about slacking on his chores	I don't have to deal with the stress of a fight with Connor. Usually I'm just tired and don't want to deal with it.	I resent picking up Connor's slack, and this creates low-level stress for me and is also bad for Connor. Doing the physical part of the extra chores increases my pain.

sleep and exercise every day. Allow the eternal to-do list to take a backseat.

You may need to have some hard conversations with family members or coworkers so that you are able to set limits, reduce your workload, and delegate in a way that supports your pain management goals.

Figure 8.2   Expense sheet: My choices

CHOICE	BENEFIT (What do I get out of it?)	PAIN COST
1.		
2.		
3.		
4.		
5.		
6.		
7.		
8.		
9.		
10		

Making Changes: Beth's Tips for Communicating with Others

Communicating with others is an important part of stress management, pain management, and self-care. Good communication gives others important context for the changes you will be making, and gives them the opportunity to understand your goals and provide support. Some conversations may be difficult, but you can set yourself up for success by using the following tips.

Tip #1: Schedule an actual meeting. Set up the day and time of the appointment to talk so people are not rushed and don't feel ambushed in the moment. Even when speaking with family, set it up in advance to create the time and space for relaxed conversation. A main goal is to ensure your audience is mentally and emotionally present. Avoid choosing a time when you know your family members are likely to be tired, hungry, or distracted.

Tip #2: Begin the conversation by telling them about your pain management and health goals. If it feels right, let family members know that your overall objective is to become healthier so that you can spend more quality time together. For instance, you may let them know that part of your medical plan is daily exercise. Over time, your daily exercise will reduce your pain and increase your physical stamina, thus allowing you to attend more family outings with them. Your loved ones are more likely to be supportive when they understand your goals and the actions related to your goals.

Tip #3: Let others know that your medical plan involves scaling back in key ways so that you can focus on self-care. If it feels right, you may wish to share with others that following your medical plan will allow you to reduce pain and medications.

Tip #4: State the specific changes you will make and how it will affect them. For example: "I will no longer be mowing the lawn, so, Connor, you will be responsible for doing that every other Saturday." Or, "I will no longer be chairing the education improvement committee, so a replacement must be found. I am happy to provide advice through emails."

Tip #5: Be clear and use specific language. Waffling and use of vague language will undermine your efforts. Be clear and specific when stating your goals, your plans, and the requests you make to others. For example: "I need to sleep well on Friday night so I have energy for the weekend. It would be great if we could eat dinner earlier, say, at 6 P.M., so I can be in bed at 9. If you can help me with the cleanup, that will help me get to bed on time, too."

Tip #6: Thank everyone for taking the time to meet with you and for supporting you in your goals. If possible, find ways to highlight the future benefits they will enjoy. ("I will be much more present on the weekends for having rested well!" Or, "Scaling back on committee work will allow me to better serve the students, and I can still provide key guidance to the group without having a leadership role.")

Tip #7: Follow through with your word. Support yourself by sticking to the commitment you made. Expect pushback from others as they test the boundaries of the new structure you set. Observe the pushback, don't take it personally even if it feels like it is, and *firmly forge ahead with your plan*. Then take delight in observing that the sky does not fall when others are disappointed or inconvenienced. Remember your goals and your commitment to yourself, and resist the temptation to rescue others from their disappointment by returning to choices that increase your pain. Remind yourself that others are capable and competent—and then step aside and allow them to demonstrate it.

Tip #8: Get help if you feel stuck. If you have ongoing difficulty making the changes that will help reduce your pain, seek the support of a psychologist to help you successfully align your choices with your goals.

Tapering Off Prescription Opioids: Tips for Success

I AM NOT A MEDICAL DOCTOR nor am I an addictionologist. As a psychologist and behaviorist, I have helped many people successfully taper off of opioids by encouraging patients to talk with their doctors about using a formula that focuses on minimizing stress on their systems. You can do specific things to help yourself successfully taper off opioids. In this chapter I provide you with basic information about ways to improve your tapering comfort and success. **Always talk to your prescribing doctor before beginning or stopping any medications—especially opioids**. Also be sure to talk with your doctor before making a change to your opioid dose.

One of the main reasons people remain on prescription opioids is that they have a natural fear of their pain worsening if they stop taking them. In fact, new research suggests that chronic pain does not worsen with opioid taper. Still, fear of worsening pain may prevent some people from even attempting an opioid taper. Once you attempt an opioid taper, having fear about your pain worsening may prevent your success with tapering. Why? Stanford researchers found that having fear of pain activates an area of your brain involved when you evaluate or regulate pain.[154]* The researchers also found that if you are sensitive to anxiety, you will tend to activate the part of the brain that looks for what's wrong—for pain.† All of this means you will be focused on your pain, and your brain will be *primed to find it and to magnify it*—this may result in your being falsely convinced that you simply cannot get off opioids.

Opioid Withdrawal Symptoms

If you take prescription opioids, you may have experienced withdrawal symptoms at some point—perhaps when you forgot to take a scheduled dose of medication. Opioid withdrawal is highly unpleasant, and for some people it feels intolerable. Anxiety, pain, shakiness, nausea, achiness—these are some of the symptoms people may experience when opioids are suddenly withdrawn. The key word here is *suddenly*. Withdrawal symptoms can be avoided if you taper slowly enough for *your body*. Common early symptoms of opioid withdrawal are shown in Table 9.1.

If you experience withdrawal symptoms, this does *not* mean that you cannot get off opioids.‡ Withdrawal symptoms mean that your opioid level was dropped too quickly and your body was surprised by the lack of medication—it did not have time to adjust. Simply that. It is physically stressful for your body to experience a sudden large drop in opioid dose—the result is withdrawal symptoms. The key is to work with your body to successfully taper your opioids—by making small changes slowly over time.

---

*The brain region is the right lateral orbital frontal cortex.

†This area is the medial prefrontal gyrus; it is involved in self-attention to one's body. www.news.stanford.edu/news/2006/february1/med-anxiety-020106.html

‡Withdrawal symptoms do not indicate addiction; in isolation, withdrawal symptoms are simply a marker of physiological dependence. Addiction involves other specific behaviors and emotions in addition to physiological dependence (see the Glossary on page 201).

Table 9.1 Common Symptoms of Opioid Withdrawal

Common early symptoms of opioid withdrawal (within 12–30 hours of last dosage)*	Common late symptoms of opioid withdrawal include
• Agitation • Anxiety • Muscle aches • Increased tearing • Insomnia • Runny nose • Sweating • Yawning • Restlessness • Opioid craving	• Abdominal cramping • Diarrhea • Dilated pupils • Goose bumps • Nausea • Vomiting

*Early symptoms of methadone withdrawal occur much later due to its long half-life.

Beth's Tips for Successful Opioid Tapering

Talk with your doctor. Always talk to your prescribing doctor before making medication changes. This is the first step in any opioid tapering program. Most doctors are happy to help their patients reduce their medications.

Timing is everything. Plan to start your taper when life is relatively calm. Wait until the timing is right. Avoid the holidays or times when work or family stress are particularly high. Remember that you want to set yourself up for success. Since stress creates challenges and worsens pain, you want to start your taper when you are *least likely* to be challenged with pain. Also, recognize that while there may never be a great time to taper, some times are definitely worse than others.

Opioids should be your only medication change during the taper. Many people fall into the trap of trying to change more than one medication at a time. They decide they will taper opioids, start an antidepressant, and go off their sleeping med all in the same month. This is a setup for failure. You will undermine your taper goals if your body is thrown into chaos with multiple changes happening at the same time. If your pain lessens, you will not know which medication change caused it, or maybe it was a combination of changes. In science, the rule is to change one thing at a time in any experiment. Think of your taper as an experiment. Then, when things are calm and you are clear about the result from that change, you can consider making changes to the next medication.

Go S-L-O-W: The turtle wins this race. Some doctors will suggest a quick taper of 1–2 weeks. *Just because you can doesn't mean you should.* By tapering slowly, you can prevent symptoms of withdrawal, stress, and anxiety. Set yourself up for success by requesting a very slow taper schedule. You may have been on opioids for 3 years. Why rush to taper off opioids in 2 weeks and risk triggering anxiety or withdrawals? Withdrawals are a sign that your system is stressed (because it is missing the opioid it expects). Stress increases pain, so this approach flies in the face of the main goal. Alternatively, you can take 2 months or more to taper and thus ensure comfort and reduced stress on your mind and body. Going slow is especially important if you have anxiety, such as panic attacks, post-traumatic stress disorder, or generalized anxiety. Ask your doctor to make small reductions (decrements) in your opioid dose about every 2 weeks. Even if you feel good, stay on a slow taper schedule and make it easy for your body.

Make ONE opioid dose change at a time. If you have been taking round-the-clock opioids, you may be on a schedule of dosing your opioids morning, midday, and bedtime. As an example, let's say you are taking 30 mg of opioids three times daily. Talk with your doctor about a taper plan that involves making small changes to *one* of the doses. You started off on 30 mg, 30 mg, 30 mg, and for your first dose reduction you may go down to 30 mg, 25 mg, 30 mg. You reduced only the midday dose, by 5 mg. When you are ready for your next dose reduction, pick

Table 9.2 An opioid dosage taper schedule

Start	30 mg	30 mg	30 mg
Week 1	30 mg	25 mg	30 mg
Week 2	30 mg	25 mg	30 mg
Week 3	25 mg	25 mg	30 mg
Week 4	25 mg	25 mg	25 mg
Week 5	25 mg	20 mg	25 mg
Week 6	20 mg	20 mg	25 mg
Week 7	20 mg	20 mg	20 mg
Week 8	20 mg	15 mg	20 mg

either the morning or the evening dose and bring that down to 25 mg. Sometimes people try to work one of the doses all the way down to zero. *Do not do this*. It is much better to keep an even opioid level in your system—as much as possible—and to slowly reduce the *overall* amount of medication. If a person gets their midday dose down to zero, they will be left with a big gap in the middle of the day with no opioid: this is likely to trigger withdrawals. Table 9.2 shows an example of keeping relatively equal opioid dosing while tapering slowly.

In 8 weeks this person reduced their daily opioid consumption by 50 percent. Notice that there is a 2-week span between the first and second dose reduction. This is the most important dose reduction because you will have a lot of anticipation. It's a good idea to go especially slowly at this very first dose reduction. **Going slowly minimizes discomfort and problems and helps you gain confidence in your ability to taper off opioids**. As you gain confidence, anxiety and stress are reduced, and you are more likely to be successful with your taper goal. Set yourself up for overall taper success by achieving success with your very first dose reduction.

This taper example is quite conservative. If you feel successful and confident after the first few dose decrements, you can speed the pace of your taper. After all, you can always drop back to the slower pace if you need to.

Use your mind-body skills. Optimize success with opioid tapering by focusing on calming your mind and body regularly throughout each day. *Calming your mind and body needs to be your main priority during the taper period.*

Watch your choices. Resist the temptation to make many life changes during your opioid taper. Wait until you are well settled into your taper or even finished with your taper before tackling new physical projects. Week 2 of your opioid taper is *not* the best time to start a home improvement project or a brand new exercise program. If you decide to taper opioids, keep the rest of your life at a constant. If you are already walking twice weekly for 30 minutes, stay with that if it is working for you. You can ramp up your activity level or make other changes once you are through with your taper.

You may need extra support. Your medical or psychological circumstances may require more structure and support. If your doctor recommends additional support, or if you are running into problems, consider working with a medical professional who can closely supervise your taper. You may be prescribed new medications to assist in the taper (e.g., Suboxone or naloxone). You may be referred to an inpatient detoxification program, or by an inpatient comprehensive pain treatment program such as the one offered by the Division of Pain Medicine at Stanford University. Within the context of opioid tapering, the purpose of these inpatient programs is often to minimize withdrawal symptoms and provide the structure and support that will best ensure your safety and success with your taper and/or medication changes.

The Unexpected Benefits of Tapering

Once you have successfully completed your opioid taper, you may be surprised by reaping a number of side benefits for your efforts.

Better Quality of Life. Recent research conducted by researchers at Boston Pain Care Center suggested that pain *does not increase during opioid taper.* At the end of their study, people taking high doses of opioids had weaned their dosage by 40 percent, had no pain increases, and had improved mood and motivation

You will learn your baseline pain level. Some people have been on opioids for many years and have no idea what their pain level would be like today without the opioids. After a slow taper, most people are surprised to learn that their pain is not as severe as they had feared or expected. In fact, *almost everyone I have worked with has reported that their pain improved as a result of adhering to their pain/stress reduction program combined with getting off opioids.* These anecdotal reports were backed up by a recently published research which similarly reported that opioid taper appears to decrease chronic pain. Once you learn your baseline pain level, you can work with your doctor to reevaluate your pain medicine strategy and needs.

After your opioid taper is complete, talk with your doctor about whether you can taper other medications. If you were prescribed medications to treat some of the side effects of opioids, you may be able to taper off of those after you are solidly through your opioid taper. Talk with your doctor.

Additional Support Resources

Addictionologists

Addictionologists are medical doctors who specialize in tapering patients off of opioids. *Working with an addictionologist does not mean you are addicted*. Your body is dependent on opioids, and for those who need extra support an addictionologist can assist with a gentle taper that avoids withdrawal symptoms. They may prescribe new medications for the taper period. Ask you doctor whether working with an addictionologist can help you successfully taper off of opioids.

However, **opioid addiction (psychological and physiological dependence)** is a clear indication that an addictionologist should be consulted. Recently, opioid dependence has been defined by the World Health Organization (WHO) as requiring the presence of a strong desire or a sense of compulsion to take the drug. For a definite diagnosis of "dependence," the WHO and DSM-V-TR* clinical guidelines require that three or more of the following six characteristic features be experienced or exhibited:

1. A strong desire or sense of compulsion to take the drug

2. Difficulties in controlling drug-taking behavior in terms of its onset, termination, or levels of use

3. A physiological withdrawal state when drug use is stopped or reduced, as evidenced by the characteristic withdrawal syndrome for the substance, or the use of the same (or a closely related) substance with the intention of relieving or avoiding withdrawal symptoms

4. Evidence of tolerance, such that increased doses of the drug are required in order to achieve effects originally produced by lower doses

5. Progressive neglect of alternative pleasures or interests either because of drug use or due to the increased amount of time necessary to obtain or take the drug or to recover from its effects

6. Persisting with drug use despite clear evidence of overtly harmful consequences, such as harm to the liver, depressive mood states, or impairment of cognitive functioning.[20]

Unlike the WHO guidelines, the DSM-V* no longer has separate diagnoses for Opioid Abuse and Opioid Dependence; they are now

---

*DSM-V-TR: Diagnostic and Statistical Manual of mental disorders, version IV, produced by the American Psychological Association, 2013

combined into a single diagnosis, Opioid Use Disorder, that is rated on a continuum from mild to severe.

Opioid Use Disorder: The DSM-V combines the DSM-IV diagnoses of Opioid Abuse and Opioid Dependence into a single disorder measured on a continuum from mild to severe. At least 2 of the following criteria are required within a 12-month period to receive a diagnosis of Opioid Use Disorder:

* Taking more opioid than intended or using for a longer period of time than intended.
* Repeated attempts to quit or control use.
* Spending a lot of time obtaining, taking, or recovering from the effects of opioids.
* Craving opioids.
* Social or interpersonal problems related to opioid use.
* Major obligations are neglected due to opioid use (e.g., work or school duties/roles).
* Giving up or reducing other activities because of opioid use.
* Using opioids even when it is physically unsafe.
* Physical or psychological problems related to opioid use.
* Tolerance for opioids.
* Withdrawal symptoms when opioids are not taken.

Inpatient Opioid Detoxification Most people are able to work with their doctors to successfully taper down opioids or get off of them completely—and this is the best route. If, however, you follow all the right steps and continue to have ongoing difficulty with your taper, you may want to talk with your doctor about inpatient opioid detox, assuming it is covered by your insurance. Inpatient detox programs provide a controlled environment, medication, and medical supervision while opioids are stopped fairly quickly—usually within days or a week. The best detox programs include multidisciplinary treatment during your stay, such as pain psychology, physical therapy, and occupational therapy.

While opioid withdrawal reactions are very uncomfortable, they are not life threatening. Recall that withdrawal symptoms are a sign that your taper is moving too fast. For a successful taper, slow down and work with your body as outlined in this chapter.

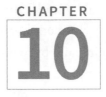

Putting It All Together: Your Empowerment Program

You have learned a lot about reducing your pain and suffering, and how to reduce your need for opioids. Knowledge is power—but only if you apply it every day. This chapter combines what you have already learned and organizes it into a practical daily plan: Your Empowerment Program.

Your empowerment program has three main strategies that will allow you to reach your goals of reduced suffering, better function, and fewer pills:

> **Strategy #1**: Lower your pain and stress responses by using techniques that condition your body and your mind.
>
> **Strategy #2**: Limit the presence of pain and stress triggers in your life.
>
> **Strategy #3**: Prevent pain flares through planning and monitoring.

Each strategy is beneficial by itself. By using just one strategy, you will make progress toward your overall goals. However, you will gain maximum control over your pain by combining the *three* strategies into your daily empowerment plan.

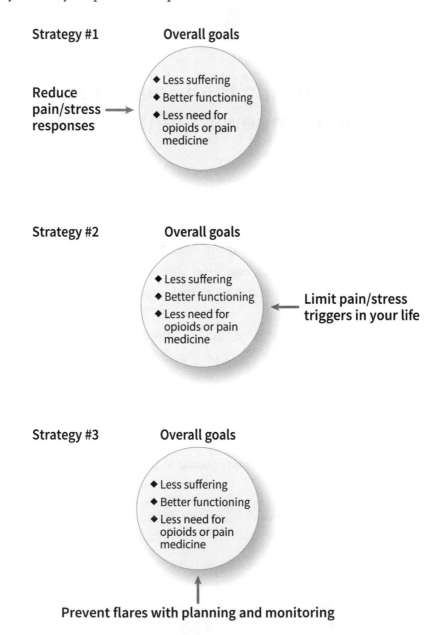

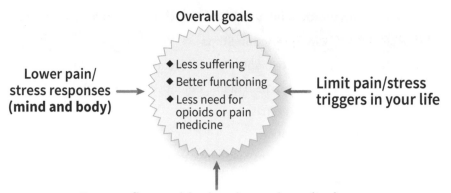

Overall goals

Lower pain/ stress responses (mind and body) → ◆ Less suffering ◆ Better functioning ◆ Less need for opioids or pain medicine ← Limit pain/stress triggers in your life

Prevent flares with planning and monitoring

When all three pathways are targeted at once, you make progress much more quickly. It's the difference between walking to your destination and taking an airplane. Moreover, using these approaches in combination will reduce your pain as much as possible. This combined approach won't just get you there more quickly; it will also help you experience less pain.

For this reason, Your Empowerment Program is designed to include all three strategies. Within each strategy you will create goals that are tailored to your life and your needs. Your plan will include specific action steps that will keep you focused on moving in the right direction. Table 10.1 on pages 180–181 outlines some sample action steps that could be included in your empowerment program. It breaks down the steps according to each of the three major strategies.

The Basic Empowerment Program: First Steps

Beginning with small goals is smart. By starting small, you have a better chance of achieving your goal. In any new program it is important to feel successful early on. When you have success at something, you want to keep doing it! You feel good about it and yourself, and you develop a positive association with the activity. The basic

Table 10.1 Example Action Steps for Each Main Strategy

Strategies	Example Action Steps
Lower My Pain/Stress Responses	• Practice diaphragmatic breathing • Listen to pain management skills audio CD • Daily exercise • Meditation • Warm baths before bedtime or during the day to help deepen my relaxation response • Prevent catastrophizing using my soother action list • Practice being gentle with myself
Limit My Pain/Stress Triggers	• Spend less time with my friend Susan (I feel depleted after our visits) • Spend more time with Jennifer, who is caring and supportive (I feel energized after I see her) • Stop "overworking" my body (at home and at the office) • Politely decline volunteering requests so I have time to take care of me • Make sleep a priority; use sleep hygiene principles with a goal of getting 8 hours of sleep nightly • Set kids up on a chore schedule with clear consequences • Every hour at work take a 3-minute break to stretch and breathe • Look into carpooling since driving increases my pain

empowerment program has fewer things to focus on each day. This may be a good formula for you. Or you may wish to focus on an even smaller program to start. You can always add more goals and steps as you move to the next level. A sample of a basic empowerment program is presented in Table 10.2 on page 182.

Strategies	Example Action Steps
Prevent My Flares	• Make pain management my number one priority
	• Spend 15 minutes each evening to take stock of my progress for the day and to review what I need to do the next day to best manage my pain/stress
	• Look ahead in my calendar to preempt future stresses (e.g., decline to attend my cousin's wedding or the family holiday dinner, or to help a friend move), and still be supportive of others without hurting myself or stressing me (e.g., send a nice gift but decline to attend the wedding, order prepared food for the holiday, etc.)

The Advanced Empowerment Program: Graduating to the Next Level

Table 10.3 on pages 186–187 presents an example of the advanced empowerment program. It is intended as a guide for your own program development. **Your Empowerment Program is a life program.** It is a commitment to yourself. Managing your pain requires you to pay exquisite attention to your choices *every day*.

More than 20 years after I was first seen in the emergency room and received opioids for my pain, I continue to make stress reduction—sensory *and* emotional stress reduction—my priority. I meditate daily and arrange my schedule to get good sleep. I have a regular exercise program that is compatible with my body's abilities. I focus on limiting my exposure to pain triggers and stress. I strive to live this program with each choice I make. **My reduced suffering did not happen by accident, and neither will yours.** Just holding the goal of reduced stress in my mind makes decision making simpler. It does not make for easy decisions, but it provides me with *clarity* about which choices I need to make to best ease stress on my system.

Table 10.2   Example Basic Empowerment Program—
Overall Goal: Reduce Suffering*

Strategies	Action Steps	M	T	W	Th	F	S	Su
Lower my pain/stress responses (mind and body)	1. Practice relaxation response 3x/day	✔	✔	2x	✔		✔	1x
	2. Listen to pain management skills CD daily	✔	✔	2x	✔	✔	2x	2x
	3. Use my catastrophizing stopper/soother list as needed (keep it handy!!)	✔			✔		✔	
Limit my pain/stress triggers	Get at least 7 hours of sleep each night (follow sleep hygiene principles)	✔		✔	✔	✔	✔	
Prevent my flares (planning and monitoring)	Each evening review my schedule for the next day. **Come into present time** and see if I need to change my schedule given how I feel (to be kinder to my body)	✔	✔		✔	✔	✔	✔

*Tapering opioids is presented here as a sample example; this may not be your goal.

Having clarity about which choices to make and actually *making* those choices are two different things. Making the right choice can be tough, even though you may clearly know what's best for you. Who really wants to get into the therapy pool at 7 A.M. instead of drinking coffee at home or staying in bed? It may seem easier to keep your mouth shut when you need to say no to your spouse or family. It may seem easier to meet your friend for lunch rather than disappoint her, even though she drains your energy and you know if you meet her you will leave feeling depleted.

The easy way is not so easy when it contributes to worsening stress. It requires discipline to follow the program when you don't want to. And it will almost certainly be disappointing to others from time to time, because you will find yourself needing to say no in order to best care for yourself. Nonetheless, keep this in mind: **When you reduce your suffering and stress, you will have more of "you" available to share with the world and those you love.**

Managing pain and reducing opioid use requires taking a hard look at the "easy" way.

Now it's time to create your own empowerment program. You can use some of the Example Action Steps listed in this chapter, or create new ones that work better for you. A sample template for documenting your plan is provided in Figure 10.1 on the next page and online at www.bullpub.com/downloads.

Beth's Tips for Success with Your Empowerment Program

Commit to making your empowerment program your number one priority. Congratulations for putting your health and well-being first! This is the only way to gain the results you desire.

Review your empowerment plan several times daily so you can see what's next on your agenda and prepare for it.

Each night create your schedule for the next day. That way you can plan for exercise and other activities, factoring in all your responsibilities. If necessary, plan your whole week in advance.

Track your progress using your empowerment log. This is important. Your memory is not a reliable gauge. Use the log to be sure you link your results to your actions.

Review your progress on your *overall goals* every 2 weeks. What do you notice? Now look at your log. Did you adhere to your action steps? First, give yourself kudos and credit for what you *did* do. You

Figure 10.1 My Empowerment Program

My Overall Goals: _____

Strategies	My Action Steps	M	T	W	Th	F	S	Su
Lower my pain/stress responses (body)								
Lower my pain/stress responses (mind)								
Limit my pain/stress triggers								
Prevent my flares (planning and monitoring)								

are making progress, and it's important to recognize and celebrate that.

Refine your action steps and goals as needed. Is there room for improvement? Were your goals too big to start? It's OK to scale back your goals. Refining your goals is not failure—it is a successful recalibration of your program. Make your goals attainable and you will succeed!

Buddy up. Stating your commitment and your goals to a friend or loved one can help you stay motivated and accountable. You can ask your friend or partner to help you stay on track by checking in with you on your progress.

Always keep an eye on your successes. Remember, whatever you choose to focus on will grow larger. If you are looking to succeed at pain management, it is important to notice what you are doing *right*. Each day, find at least one positive thing you did toward your empowerment program (e.g., "I caught myself catastrophizing and stopped it in the first 5 minutes"). Notice your small successes and celebrate them! It's the accumulation of small successes that will allow you to realize your big goal.

Don't stay stuck. If you find yourself struggling to make progress even after scaling back your goals and action steps, seek help. Work with a health coach, counselor, therapist, or psychologist. Find a therapist who specializes in cognitive behavioral therapy to help you dissolve roadblocks and keep you moving forward.

I Am in a Pain Flare. Now What?

Part of your empowerment program is preventing pain flares. Let's talk more about what to do when a pain flare happens. I've talked about this in earlier chapters, but it bears a focused discussion here so you can think about integrating it into your overall plan.

When you are in a pain flare, dealing with your pain and discomfort becomes your priority. The pitfall is focusing on the pain instead

Table 10.3 Advanced Empowerment Program—Overall Goals: Reduce Suffering, Improve Functioning, Reduce Medication

Strategies	Action Steps	M	T	W	Th	F	S	Su
Lower my pain/stress responses (body)	1. Practice relaxation response 3x/day	✔			✔	✔		
	2. Listen to pain management skills CD daily	✔	✔		✔	✔	✔	
	3. Exercise—pool class (W, F); walk 25 min 2x/week at lunchtime	✔	✔	✔	✔	✔		
Lower my pain/stress responses (mind)	1. Practice thought monitoring	✔	✔	✔	✔	✔	✔	✔
	2. Use my catastrophizing stopper/soother list as needed (keep a copy at home and in my car!)	✔	✔	2x	✔	✔	✔	2x
	3. Practice being gentle with myself	✔	✔	✔		✔	✔	2x
Limit my pain/stress triggers	1. Schedule family meeting; discuss goals		✔					
	2. Delegate 1/3 of house chores to create time to exercise				✔			✔
	3. Sleep alone 2x/week to ensure better sleep		✔		✔			
	4. Work with counselor to figure out how to end friendships that are draining	✔				✔		

of *learning* from the pain flare. Often a pain flare has a rich story to tell. A pain flare contains information about you, and if you take time to learn from it, you will be prepared to prevent future pain flares.

Donna learned how to reclaim her power by investigating her pain flares.

Strategies	Action Steps	M	T	W	Th	F	S	Su
Prevent my flares (planning and monitoring)	1. Each evening review my schedule for the next day. **Evaluate** whether I need to change my schedule given how I feel in the moment. Give myself permission to modify again in the morning if I have not slept well that night	✔	✔	✔	✔	✔	✔	✔
	2. Let family know Thanksgiving will not be hosted at our house this year—too stressful!!				✔			✔

❧   ❧

Donna's Story

Donna arrived at my office on a Monday, moving slowly. "I am having a horrible pain day," she muttered as she sat down. "I almost didn't come here today. I wanted to call and cancel. I wonder if I can get an increase in my medication just to get me through this. Do you know if Dr. Richards is in the clinic today?"

I skirted the focus on medication because I knew it was not the best place to start. "Of course you wanted to cancel," I empathized. "You are suffering. Good for you for getting yourself here today. That took real dedication."

Then I asked her the magic question. "So what did you do this weekend?"*

---

*If I had seen her on Thursday, I would have asked her what she had been doing 1–3 days before her pain flare.

She paused and then described how on Saturday she and her husband, John, drove 2½ hours to another city to help a friend move. Helping the friend involved some light lifting and being on her feet for about 5 hours. Then there was the 2½-hour drive home.

Sounds simple enough, but Donna was quite debilitated from her fibromyalgia. Before we started working together, she spent many of her days in bed. *All* day in bed. She had made great progress and was becoming more active, but 5 hours of driving, 5 hours on her feet, and lifting boxes (no matter how light) was asking too much of her body. She was not used to that level of activity.

I knew Donna well enough to know that she could handle very direct feedback from me. "Of course you have a pain flare!" I said irreverently after she explained her weekend activities. "That was quite the activity binge for you." Donna nodded. "I guess it was."

"It makes sense, doesn't it? Your body is just sending you some information here. What do you think you body is trying to tell you?" "That it was too much," she said.

"OK, your body is just trying to get your attention. And it definitely got your attention with the pain. So knowing this—if you could rewind the tape and start over, what would you do differently?"

"I guess I would need to tell Joann that I couldn't help her move," she said. "But that would be hard to do. I feel obligated as her friend. Plus, she helped us when we moved."

"Yes, that makes good sense. Of course you want to help Joann. Your heart is in the right place. But your body isn't on board. Your body has some real limitations. Would it help if you talked about those limitations with Joann?" "Maybe," Donna replied.

I coached Donna to do three things. First, it's always easier to discuss things well in advance of the actual event. The moment Joann asks Donna to help with the move is the best time to bring it up.

Second, I coached Donna to tell Joann the truth: She wants to help her. She would love to help with the move. She feels indebted because

Joann has been such a helpful friend in the past and she wants to return the favor.

Third, and most importantly, we talked about the importance of being honest about her pain. For example: "As much as I want to help I'm afraid my medical condition won't allow it. But I would love to support you in another way. John can absolutely help with the move, but I will stay home. I am wondering if I could help hire someone else to help you. Or I can send John over with lunch so you don't have to worry about food during the move."

It's true this doesn't always work smoothly. Donna found that she had to let at least one friendship go because the friend pushed back and was dismissive of Donna's need for self-care. Donna came to realize it wasn't much of a friendship. "Now I feel good about having people in my life who are truly supporting me," she said.

ಇ   ✄

Ultimately, it was important for Donna to understand the connection between her pain flares and her choices. That way she could begin changing her choices to reduce her pain flares. By doing so, she would reduce her use of pain medication. By unveiling the "mystery" of her pain, she learned she had more control than she thought.

To be sure, some pain flares are random. The pain comes from nowhere and is not related to any decision you made or action you took. But when a pain flare happens, *you owe it to yourself to do a small investigation.* By investigating your pain flare, you will learn as much as possible so that you become as empowered as possible.

Pain flare summary:

1. Pain flares contain information.

2. By collecting information about your pain flare and what happened in the days prior to it, you can learn about your pain triggers.

3. Learning from your pain flares will help you lessen and prevent future pain flares and reduce use of pain medication.

Beth's Steps for Investigating Your Pain Flare

Step 1: Think about what you did in the days before your pain flare started. Can you make a connection between anything you did? Overwork? Change in habits, medication, or sleep? Was it a particularly stressful time for you? Was anything *different* in the days that preceded your pain increase?

Very often, people are able to identify something different that happened (or that they did) that is a likely explanation for the pain flare. If you are able to source a likely cause of your pain flare, go on to the next step of investigation.

Step 2: Ask yourself the following questions:

- If I could rewind the past 1 to 3 days, what could I do differently to prevent my pain flare or reduce it?

- Am I willing to make different choices in the future to lessen my pain flares and need for pain medication?

- What do I need to do *now* in order to set myself up for future success with reducing my pain flares? (Integrate this into My Empowerment Program).

Donna discovered that what she needed to do *now* was talk to her husband and later to her friend. She needed to catch them both up to speed about her limitations, and how her choices impacted her pain. Donna chose to have simple conversations where she said, "I'm realizing I can't do all the things I want to do. It's frustrating because I *want* to do more, and I want to do more for other people, but I can see that it's easier to work *with* my body rather than fight against my limitations. I guess that means I will be doing less in the future, but the good news is that by doing less, I will also have fewer 'down' days and pain flares."

Importantly, Donna stopped focusing on how her medications could "fix" her pain flares and instead began focusing on how she could *prevent* the pain flares in the first place. She found this shift in focus empowering, as it put *her—not her medications*—in the driver's seat of her pain management.

Use the template provided in Figure 10.4 below (and online at www.bullpub.com/downloads) to conduct your own investigation of your pain flares.

Figure 10.4   My pain flare investigation

1. What is my pain flare telling me?	
2. Was anything different in the days that preceded my pain flare?	
3. What would help reduce future pain flares?	
4. What can I do now to set myself up for success with preventing future pain flares?	
5. Do I need extra support in making changes?	

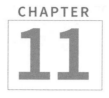

An Example of Mindful Use of Prescription Opioids

IF YOU CHOOSE TO MAKE OPIOIDS ONE PART of your pain care plan, you can apply the information and tools you have learned to use them mindfully.

It is useful to take a step back and broadly consider two vastly different approaches to treating pain: the purely pill-based approach* and the comprehensive approach.† To illustrate this point, consider two people, Luis and Robert. Both have chronic back pain, but their pain is treated differently. Luis's treatment approach is focused on pills alone, whereas Robert receives a treatment focused on mindful use and self-empowerment. As you can see from Table 11.1 on pages 194–195, they have vastly different outcomes.

In the example, Luis receives a pill bottle alone while Robert receives comprehensive pain care. Notice how the comprehensive approach empowers Robert while Luis remains dependent on a prescription for pain relief.

---

*In the case of opioids and many other pain medications, there is limited evidence to support the value of a purely pill-based treatment approach.

†Research shows that comprehensive care is the best treatment approach for various types of chronic pain.

Table 11.1 Contrasting Approaches to Pain Treatment

	Luis: Prescription Only	**Robert: Multidisciplinary/ Comprehensive Care***
What the doctor provides	• Opioids	• Opioids • Referral to physical therapy • Referral to pool therapy • Referral to pain psychology • Education about pain and the benefit of multidisciplinary care • Education about the limitations of opioids • A requirement of smoking cessation if opioids will be continued (resources given) • Hormone testing
What happens at follow-up visits	• Refills	Focus is on achieving the goals Robert created: • To better manage stress (psychology) • To practice better **pacing** with activities (psychology and physical therapy) • To increase exercise and endurance (physical therapy) • To improve sleep using sleep hygiene principles (psychology and physician visit) Medical follow-up also includes monitoring for opioid risks/side effects.

*Notably, "comprehensive" pain care is a health care bargain because education, psychology, physical therapy and other so-called conservative, ancillary, and behaviorally focused treatments are cheap in comparison to allopathic medicine and interventions. Ultimately, the best bargain is the treatment that works, and this is most often a combination of approaches—multidisciplinary pain care.

	Luis: Prescription Only	Robert: Multidisciplinary/ Comprehensive Care*
The message being sent by the doctor	Your pain is only helped by pills.	• Opioids are one part of your overall plan. • Opioids are helpful only to the extent that they allow you to fully engage in your comprehensive plan. • You will earn good outcomes by engaging in your pain care and making life changes.
What is learned (thoughts)	My pain is something that just happens and I have little control over it other than taking medicine.	I can control my pain through exercise and stress management techniques, setting good limits with other people, taking excellent care of myself. My choices impact my pain, so I focus on making choices that help my pain—that way I can keep my opioid dose as low as possible.
What is learned (emotions)	I feel anxious about not having my medication; I need to have my prescription in my possession to feel calm.	I feel confident in my ability to manage pain without the medication. Sure, the medication helps, but I'm the one who controls the "volume dial" on my pain.
What is learned (actions)	My actions and choices are ignorable when it comes to my pain.	When I engage in my pain care plan, I feel better. My actions directly impact my pain, and therefore I make choices that help me feel good.

Now imagine that Luis and Robert experience severe financial strain—a common and very stressful circumstance. Severe stress is likely to cause various problems, such as increased muscle tension, sleeplessness, and anxiety—all things that worsen pain. Robert has learned many ways to manage his pain. He has been exercising because he learned it is one of the best treatments for pain. It turns out that exercise also helps decrease worry, anxiety, and muscle tension, and it improves sleep. Furthermore, Robert has been calming his nervous system regularly with relaxation therapy, so his pain is lower to begin with, and his mind is calmer and better able to handle the financial stress.

Luis, on the other hand, has no techniques to manage his pain or this new stress. His pain was high to begin with, but now with the financial problem he finds his pain is even worse. He calls his doctor complaining of more pain and asks if he can get an increase in his opioids to help bring his pain back down. His doctor determines that indeed he has legitimate increased pain and that he has never lost a prescription or exhibited other "red flag" behaviors, so he agrees to increase his opioids. They set a follow-up appointment for 3 months from now.

Fortunately, you will never be subject to Luis's fate, even if a past doctor has treated your pain with pills alone. You have read this book and you know better now. You have developed your own empowerment plan and have a road map for how to get your life back. You know that your control does not lie in a pill bottle. For some people, mindful use of opioids is an important part of their pain care plan. For others, avoiding opioids is desirable or essential. It's up to you to weigh your risks and benefits, to discuss them with your doctor, and to arrive at a decision that's comfortable for you. Empowered pain care begins by making an informed choice about opioids. Your empowered pain management is then *lived each day* through your good choices and excellent self-care.

Appendix: Historical Notes

In response to the growing US painkiller crisis, the Obama administration in the spring of 2011 called for tighter legislation surrounding physicians' privileges for prescribing opioids. The proposed legislation required physicians to receive specific training before being allowed to prescribe opioids.[155]

Physician groups such as the American Academy of Family Physicians (AAFP) opposed the legislation—not in principle but in practice. The AAFP argued that additional opioid education would burden physicians, and therefore fewer physicians would be willing to prescribe opioids. They warned that the opioid education requirement would cause a shortage of doctors willing and able to prescribe opioids for pain patients. The physician lobbyist group's arguments were successful, and in July 2012 the proposed legislation was defeated. The federal government would not mandate that physicians receive any special training prior to prescribing opioids.*

Still, with no immediate consensus on national solutions, alarm was building.

"The problem of opioid abuse is bad and getting worse," remarked Senator Charles E. Grassley. Senator Max Baucus, chairman of the Finance Committee, went further by declaring that "overdoses on narcotic painkillers have become epidemic, and it's becoming clear that patients aren't getting a full and clear picture of the risks posed

---

*However, certain states—such as California—have laws that require physicians to receive opioid education prior to prescribing.

by their medications." Calls for inquiry and change were growing louder.

In May of 2012 Senators Grassley and Baucus opened an investigation into the national opioid crisis. One goal of the investigation was to understand to what extent financial ties between doctors and pharmaceutical companies were influencing treatment practices and opioid prescribing patterns. Theirs was not the first congressional investigation.

A 2003 congressional investigation revealed that the opioid epidemic was partially and significantly related to the fact that pharmaceutical companies marketed false information about the safety and efficacy of opioids and engaged in illegal marketing practices. Purdue Pharma, in particular, targeted both doctors and patients in their marketing campaigns to encourage the use of OxyContin.* Pharmaceutical companies engaged in dangerous marketing campaigns that grossly overstated the benefits of opioids while downplaying the risks, thus setting up patients and doctors for a tidal wave of problems. For instance, it was widely stated that only 1 percent of people prescribed opioids for chronic pain would become addicted—a statement based on no credible data whatsoever. Thousands of patients and doctors would discover the truth the hard way. By 2001 OxyContin became the most prescribed brand-name narcotic medication in the United States.

---

*OxyContin is Purdue Pharma's brand name for time-release oral oxycodone. OxyContin is an opioid narcotic, schedule II drug originally approved by FDA in 1995 for the treatment of moderate-to-severe pain lasting more than a few days, as indicated in the original label. Oxycodone, the active ingredient in OxyContin, is a compound that is similar to morphine and is also found in oxycodone-combination pain relief drugs such as Percocet, Percodan, and Tylox. Because of its controlled-release property, OxyContin contains more active ingredient and needs to be taken less often (twice a day) than these other oxycodone-containing drugs. FDA approved the revised OxyContin label in July 2001 to describe the time frame as "when a continuous around-the-clock analgesic is needed for an extended period of time." (sourced from the 2003 GAO report)

The pharmaceutical industry benefited financially by promoting bad pain treatment practices that ultimately ended up harming and killing patients.* Following federal prosecution in 2007, Purdue Pharma, the Purdue president, the chief medical officer, and the primary attorney all pleaded guilty to misleading the public about OxyContin's risk for addiction. The company was fined for falsely marketing OxyContin as being less addictive and less subject to abuse than other pain medications. But the damage was done. Opioid prescribing patterns continue to rise each year, with patients and prescribers believing in each case that they are indicated, safe, and effective.

Public awareness of the issue was fueled further by the high-profile prescription opioid–related deaths of celebrities such as Brittany Murphy† and Heath Ledger.‡ Awareness was also raised by many people having some personal connection with opioids: either they had chronic pain themselves and were taking opioids, or a friend or family member had chronic pain or opioid abuse issues. Communities were being affected. Kids were reporting that it was alarmingly easy for them to purchase prescription opioids from dealers. High school kids were buying OxyContin at school, taking it at parties, and dying from overdose. The prescription opioid deaths that were mushrooming across the nation became regular front-page news.

What had become front-page news and a governmental priority was in fact old news to those of us treating people with chronic pain.

---

*For a detailed investigative report on how the pharmaceutical industry's marketing practices fueled the pain killer trap is the U.S. the reader is referred to the 2003 book by Barry Meier of The New York Times, entitled *Pain Killer: A "wonder" drug's trail of addiction and death*. (USA: Rodale).

†Murphy's death was ruled to be from the combined effects of acetaminophen and hydrocodone (components of her Vicodin prescription) and a respiratory infection (acute pneumonia).

‡Ledger died from a combination of the opioids oxycodone, hydrocodone, and the benzodiazepines diazepam (brand name: Valium), and alprazolam (brand name: Xanax), among others.

Particularly since 2005, for people with chronic pain taking prescription opioids, the opioids and problems related to them seemed to absorb much of the medical visit.[39]

National Law Passed to Improve the Safety of Prescription Opioids

On July 9, 2012, the FDA approved the risk evaluation and mitigation strategy (REMS) for opioids that fall under the category of "extended release" or "long acting" (e.g., OxyContin, Avinza, Opana ER, MS Contin, Palladone, Nucynta ER, Kadian, Exalgo, Duragesic [fentanyl], Butrans, and methadone). The REMS plan required that as of 2013 the manufacturers of long-acting opioids provide safety information to prescribers, make online continuing education available to prescribers, and provide safety information to patients in handout format. REMS focuses on the abuse, resale, and overdose risks. While REMS requires the information on risks be made *available*, the defeat of the broader legislation means that prescribers are *not required* to complete specific opioid continuing education in order to prescribe the medications.

It is expected that improved training will reduce opioid prescribing and bring greater attention to the potential harms of opioids, and will reduce opioid-related deaths. REMS is a good first step in addressing one part of the opioid prescribing problem.

The larger issue remains: people need access to pain care that empowers *them* to reduce their suffering. Empowerment from pain does not come in a bottle. **Instead of national initiatives that focus on opioid legislation and opioid dose limitations, I dream of a national health care initiative aimed at giving the *people with chronic pain* the tools to control their pain experience, their health, and their lives.** Such a pain care initiative may be far down the road. In the meantime, I hope this book helps you reclaim your control from pain and pills, so that you are able to live your best life possible.

Glossary

Abuse, opioid (DSM-IV definition): *See* "Opioid Use Disorder" as it is now classified in the DSM-V.

Addiction: A chronic, relapsing disease characterized by compulsive drug seeking and use, despite harmful consequences, and by neurochemical and molecular changes in the brain.

Addictionologist: (1) A medical doctor who is board eligible or certified by the American Society of Addiction Medicine and who specializes in diagnosing and managing patients with addiction disorders.
(2) A health professional (e.g., a psychiatrist) who manages a patient with dependence on various substances of abuse (e.g., alcohol, cocaine, opiates, tobacco).

Analgesia: Absence of pain in response to stimulation that would normally be painful. Pain medication provides analgesia—the absence of pain (or more accurately, the reduction of pain).

Barbiturate: A class of drugs that depress the central nervous system, cause relaxation and sleepiness, and are commonly prescribed as a sedative or hypnotic. Barbiturates and opioids both cause central nervous system depression and are dangerous when taken together, as respiratory depression and death may result.

Benzodiazepine: A class of drugs that depress the central nervous system and cause relaxation. Historically, they have been used to treat anxiety, although they are not the best treatment and long-term use should be avoided due to risk for physiological and psychological dependence. Benzodiazepines and opioids are both central nervous system depressants and therefore should not be taken together except in rare circumstances due to the risk of death from respiratory depression. If you are prescribed benzodiazepines and opioids speak with your doctor to understand the rationale and the risks. Ask about other ways to manage your symptoms that carry less risk.

Breakthrough pain: Pain that comes on suddenly for short periods of time and is not alleviated by the patient's normal pain suppression management. The concept of breakthrough pain originated in cancer pain treatment. The notion of breakthrough pain in non-cancer chronic pain is flawed because it is predicated on the notion that it is possible—indeed, expected—that patients are pain-free because of their pain medication, and that "breakthrough pain" should be erradicated with more medication. In terms of the goal of minimizing opioid use, in my clinical experience I find it it may be particularly useful to examine the role of one's choices as a precipitant to pain "breaking through" the normal dose of medication.

Buprenorphine: A semisynthetic opioid medication approved by the FDA in October 2002 for treatment of opioid addiction. Suboxone is a formulation widely used for opioid addiction or for weaning off opioids. Temgesic is a sublingual tablet used for moderate to severe pain; Norspan and Butrans are transdermal preparations used for chronic pain.

Catastrophizing: A psychological experience regarding pain that includes being unable to focus on anything else but the pain (rumination), magnification of pain, and feeling helpless about pain.Pain catastrophizing is one of the most powerful predictors of pain suffering and the pain experience.

Central nervous system (CNS): The brain and spinal cord.

Cognitive behavioral therapy (CBT): A theoretical orientation in clinical psychology that focuses on helping clients achieve goals and reduce symptoms and distress by changing cognitive and emotional processes and behaviors in the "here and now." CBT is an evidence-based psychotherapeutic approach most widely used in the psychological treatment of chronic pain.

Cortisol: A stress hormone produced by the adrenal glands released during physical and emotional stress. Cortisol prevents the release of substances in the body that cause inflammation. It is common for people with chronic pain to have low levels of cortisol (hypocortisolemia), sometimes called adrenal exhaustion. Low cortisol leaves a person more vulnerable to the effects of stress and inflammation. This is one reason why it is critical that people with chronic pain best manage stress in their lives.

CT scan: Computerized tomography (CT), which uses X-rays to image structures in the body.

Delirium: Rapid onset confusion and disorientation that can be caused by opioids or other medications. Elderly people are at particular risk for opioid-related delirium and falls related to an acute change in mental status.

Dependence, opioid: Whereas the DSM-IV had separate diagnostic categories for Opioid Abuse and Opioid Dependence, the DSM-V merges both into "Opioid Use Disorder."

Diaphragmatic breathing: A therapeutic breathing technique, also known as abdominal breathing, which uses the diaphragm, a large muscle located between the chest and the abdomen, and causes the abdomen to expand with each breath. This causes a negative pressure within the chest, forcing air into the lungs. The negative pressure also pulls blood into the chest, improving the return of blood to the heart. Diaphragmatic breathing can be learned and is an excellent tool to stimulate the relaxation response, which results in less tension and an overall sense of well-being.

Diversion: The transfer of a controlled substance from a lawful to an unlawful channel of distribution or use (Source: Section 309, Diversion Prevention and Control Uniform Controlled Substances Act, National Conference of Commissioners on Uniform State Laws, 1994). In the case of opioids, diversion often involves patients selling or giving others opioids prescribed to them. Dr. David Joranson provides an excellent presentation on diversion and balancing roles of the clinician and law enforcement at www.painpolicy.wisc.edu/domestic/Diversion_slides.pdf.

fMRI: Functional magnetic resonance imaging, which measures brain activity by detecting associated changes in blood flow.

Function: In chronic pain, the level of daily physical activation and capacity.

Functional goals: Concrete, measurable activities. Examples include walking a mile every day, doing home exercises daily, practicing relaxation twice a day, pacing housework on the weekends, sleeping 7 hours nightly, socializing once weekly.

Homeostasis: The tendency of an organism or a cell to regulate its internal conditions, usually by a system of feedback controls, so as to stabilize health and functioning, regardless of the outside changing conditions (Source: Biology-Online.org/dictionary).

Hyperalgesia: An increased response to a stimulus that is normally painful. E.g., experiencing severe pain in a situation that would normally cause mild or moderate pain.

Iatrogenic: From the Greek *iatros*, meaning "doctor" or "healer," and *gennan*, meaning "as a result." (Source: About.com). Iatrogenic injury may be a form of unintended medical error, or it may simply be a consequence of medical treatment (e.g., side effects that then require de novo treatment). Some of the iatrogenic risks of long-term opioid use include endocrinopathy (disturbed hormones in men and women), reduced fertility, and sleep disturbance.

Inflammation: Typically, a localized protective reaction of tissue to irritation, injury, or infection, characterized by pain, redness, swelling, and sometimes loss of function. Systemic inflammation is mediated by the immune system and is the result of release of proinflammatory cytokines from immune-related cells. Systemic inflammation is measurable in blood or plasma. Inflammatory factors appear to play a role in the transition of acute pain to the chronic state. Inflammatory factors are also involved in the stress response. Multiple independent studies have shown that psychological stress triggers the release of proinflammatory factors into the bloodstream (often referred to as *systemic inflammation*).

Lamaze: Relating to or being a method of childbirth that involves psychological and physical preparation by the mother in order to suppress pain and facilitate delivery without drugs (Source: *Merriam-Webster*). A main Lamaze technique involves diaphragmatic breathing to reduce psychological and physical stress.

Long-acting opioids: Sustained release formulations of opioid medications that reduce fluctuations of analgesic blood level and require less frequent dosing.

Malinger: To pretend or exaggerate illness or incapacity in order to gain something (called *secondary gain*), such as workers' compensation, sympathy, disability leave, or prescription opioids.

Morphine: An alkaloid narcotic drug extracted from opium; a powerful, habit-forming narcotic used to relieve pain.

Narcotic: A drug (as opium or morphine) that in moderate doses dulls the senses, relieves pain, and induces profound sleep, but in excessive doses causes stupor, coma, or convulsions (Source: *Merriam-Webster*).

Neuropathic pain: Pain initiated or caused by a primary lesion or dysfunction in the nervous system.

Norepinephrine: A neurotransmitter present in some areas of the brain and the adrenal glands; decreases smooth muscle contraction and increases heart rate; often released in response to low blood pressure or stress.

Noxious: Interpretation of a stimulus as being an actual or potential tissue-damaging event (e.g., if you place your hand on a hot burner, you would perceive the burner to be a noxious stimulus.

Opiates: Naturally occurring alkaloids in the opium poppy plant. The term *opiate* is often used incorrectly to describe opioids, drugs that have opium- or morphine-like pharmacological action.

Opioids: Controlled drugs or narcotics most often prescribed for the management of pain; natural or synthetic chemicals based on opium's active component (morphine) that work by mimicking the actions of pain-relieving chemicals produced in the body.

Opioid Use Disorder: The DSM-V combines the DSM-IV diagnoses of Opioid Abuse and Opioid Dependence into a single disorder measured on a continuum from mild to severe. At least 2 of the following criteria are required within a 12-month period to receive a diagnosis of Opioid Use Disorder:

- Taking more opioid than intended or using for a longer period of time than intended.
- Repeated attempts to quit or control use.
- Spending a lot of time obtaining, taking, or recovering from the effects of opioids.
- Craving opioids.
- Social or interpersonal problems related to opioid use.
- Major obligations are neglected due to opioid use (e.g., work or school duties/roles).
- Giving up or reducing other activities because of opioid use.
- Using opioids even when it is physically unsafe.

- Physical or psychological problems related to opioid use.
- Tolerance for opioids.
- Withdrawal symptoms when opioids are not taken.

Opiophobia: A health care provider's fear that patients will become addicted to opioids even when using them appropriately; can lead to the underprescribing of opioids for pain management.

Pacing: Balanced, mindful engagement in activity. Pacing requires rest breaks be built into activities, which allow for recovery and a chance to assess how your body feels. A main goal of pacing is to slowly build endurance without causing pain flares.

Pain: An unpleasant sensory and emotional experience associated with actual or potential tissue damage or described in terms of such damage (Source: International Association for the Study of Pain).

Painkiller: Commonly defined as any medication used to treat pain. Within the context of this book, *painkiller* is used to refer to opioid-derived drugs only (e.g., fentanyl, Vicodin, Percocet, oxycodone, OxyContin) and not other types of pain medications, such as ibuprofen or aspirin.

Pain psychology: A discipline within the field of psychology focused specifically on helping people with chronic pain. A pain psychologist typically holds a doctoral degree in psychology and has completed a 1- or 2-year fellowship in either pain or health psychology. Pain psychology is largely based on cognitive behavioral principles and helps people learn ways to better self-manage pain and the factors that influence pain. Sessions may include pain education, pain management skill building, stress management, and learning to shift expectations. Specific goals are crafted to meet the needs of each individual.

Pain threshold: The least experience of pain that a person can recognize.

Pain tolerance level: The greatest level of pain that a person can tolerate.

Perception: Physical sensation interpreted in light of experience. Pain perception is the interpretation of pain, as seen through the lens of one's experience.

Physical dependence: An adaptive physiological state that can occur with regular drug use and results in withdrawal when drug use is discontinued. (Physical dependence alone is not the same as addiction, which involves compulsive drug seeking and use, despite its harmful consequences.)

Prescription drug abuse: The intentional misuse of a medication outside of the normally accepted standards of its use.

Prescription drug misuse: Taking a medication in a manner other than that prescribed or for a different condition than that for which the medication is prescribed.

Pseudoaddiction: Drug-seeking behavior that simulates real addiction, thought to occur in patients who are receiving inadequate pain control. However, this remains a controversial topic, with some experts believing there are no good data to support the term.

Respiratory depression: Depression of respiration (breathing) that results in the reduced availability of oxygen to vital organs.

Sedatives: Drugs that suppress anxiety and relax muscles; the National Survey on Drug Use and Health classification includes benzodiazepines, barbiturates, and other types of CNS depressants.

Short-acting opioids: Opioids with a very short half-life. Patients who use short-acting opioids often dose several times daily and are more likely to have variable analgesia. Short-acting opioids have a greater potential for abuse.

Stimulants: Drugs that increase or enhance the activity of monamines (such as dopamine and norepinephrine) in the brain, which leads to increased heart rate, blood pressure, and respiration; used to treat only a few disorders, such as narcolepsy and ADHD.

Stress: In this book I refer to stress using the basic definition of disruption in equilibrium or well-being—what is classically known as homeostasis. Anything that causes a "disequilibrium" is considered a stressor. For instance, sleep deprivation is stressful and taxing on the human body—it is a disequilibrium in homeostasis, the point of balance considered optimal for an individual's health and wellbeing. The experience of stress leads to changes in the brain, body, and behavior as an individual attempts to either correct the disequilibrium or adapt to it.

Chronic pain is one form of chronic stress—experienced as a disequilibrium in comfort that is associated with changes in neural responses, neuromuscular patterns, behavior, biochemical responses, psychological responses, sleep—all of which have a profound influence on global health. Chronic stress is a known precursor to disease.

Suboxone: A semisynthetic opioid (*see* buprenorphine).

Tolerance: A condition in which higher doses of a drug are required to produce the same effects as experienced initially.

Urine drug screen (UDS): Often used by clinics or opioid prescribers to ensure (1) that the prescribed opioid is in the patient's system and (2) that no illicit drugs are being used. If a UDS shows a prescribed opioid is missing from a patient's urine, the provider has evidence to suggest the opioids are being diverted and potentially sold illegally.

Withdrawal: A variety of symptoms that occur after chronic use of some drugs is reduced or stopped. These symptoms may include shaking, sweating, craving, sleeplessness, achiness, nausea, anxiety, restlessness, and extreme discomfort (*see* dependence). The goal of detoxification is the amelioration of withdrawal symptoms.

Resources

Locating a Pain Physician
American Academy of Pain Physicians (www.painmed.org).

Locating a Board-Certified Pain Physician
Pain physicians are certified by the American Board of Anesthesiology. Pain medicine is a specialty board certification. To begin your search, visit the main site at www.directory.theaba.org and choose "Search Physician Directory" and select "Pain Medicine" from the drop down menu.

Locating a Multidisciplinary Pain Clinic
Multidisciplinary pain clinics are often linked to university medical schools. A few examples include the Pain Management Center at Stanford University, the University of California San Diego Center for Pain Medicine, the Pain Management Center at Brigham and Women's Hospital in Boston, and the various pain clinic offerings at the University of Michigan. Search the Internet to see if there is a multidisciplinary pain clinic in your area.

Locating a Pain Psychologist
Pain psychologists are most easily found in multidisciplinary pain clinic settings. Pain psychologists typically have a PhD (or PsyD) in clinical psychology and postdoctoral training in pain management. V.A. hospitals typically have health psychologists on staff who specialize in chronic pain. Some pain psychologists have private practices in the community. Finding a community psychologist who specializes in pain may require some searching. Here are some tips:

1. Ask your doctor if he/she is aware of a good local pain psychologist.
2. If you live in the 13-state region of the western United States (AZ, CA, WA, OR, UT, MT, NM, CO, HI, ID, WY, AK, NV), you

may search the website of the Western Pain Society (www.western-painsociety.org/directory). If you live in Oregon, the Pain Society of Oregon also offers a similar search feature (www.painsociety.com).

3. You may do a simple Google search of the term "pain psychologist" and your city. Community psychologists often have websites that you can visit to learn more about them.

4. *Psychology Today* has an online therapist directory with profiles attached. You can read about the therapist's background and their specialty and approach. Be sure to look for therapists that use a cognitive behavioral treatment approach, as this is best for pain.

Pain News

National Pain Report (www.nationalpainreport.com).

Chronic Pain Advocacy Groups

* American Chronic Pain Association (www.theacpa.org). Check the ACPA website for details about free support groups in your area.

* American Pain Society (www.ampainsoc.org/resources). The APS website has links of resources for people in pain and for providers.

* American Academy of Pain Medicine (www.painmed.org/patient-center/main.aspx). This link to the AAPM Patient Center offers information about pain, pain treatment, and various resources.

* Arthritis Foundation (www.arthritis.org).

* The Vulvar Pain Foundation (www.thevpfoundation.org).

* American Council for Headache Education (www.achenet.org).

* Cancer Care (www.cancercare.org).

* For Grace (Empowering Women in Pain at www.forgrace.org/women/in/pain_home).

Sleep

Sleep hygiene education from the National Sleep Foundation (www.sleepfoundation.org/article/ask-the-expert/sleep-hygiene).

Books

Living a Healthy Life with Chronic Conditions: Self-Management of Heart Disease, Arthritis, Diabetes, Depression, Asthma, Bronchitis, Emphysema and Other Physical and Mental Health Conditions, 4th edition (Kate Lorig et al. 2012) (www.bullpub.com).

Also available as:

Audiobook: *Living a Healthy Life with Chronic Conditions*, 4th edition (audiobook, CD)

Canadian edition: *Living a Healthy Life with Chronic Conditions*, 4th edition (for ongoing physical and mental health conditions)

Spanish edition: *Tomando control de su salud: Una guía para el manejo de las enfermedades del corazón, diabetes, asma, bronquitis, enfisema y otros problemas crónicos*, 4th edition

French edition: *Vivre en santé : Autogestion des cardiopathies, de l'arthrite, du diabète, de la dépression, de l'asthme, de la bronchite, de l'emphysème et d'autres maladies physiques et mentales*, 4th edition

Additional Audio CDs

Enhanced Pain Management: Binaural Relaxation, © 2013, audio CD / audiofile by Beth Darnall, PhD is available for individual purchase at www.bullpub.com

Pain Management Skills CD, © 2013, (Beth Darnall, PhD, 2010)

www.bethdarnall.com; see "Products" tab

Relaxation for Mind and Body: Pathways to Healing (Catherine Regan, PhD, and Rick Seidel, PhD, 2012 at www.bullpub.com).

References

1. IMS Institute for Healthcare Informatics, *The Use of Medicines in the United States: Review of 2011*, 2012.

2. CDC, Vital Signs: Overdoses of prescription opioid pain relievers and other drugs among women—United States, 1999–2010, in *Morbidity and Mortality Weekly Report*, 2013, Centers for Disease Control: Atlanta, GA. p. 537–42.

3. Mezei, L., and B.B. Murinson, Pain education in North American medical schools. *J Pain*, 2011. **12**(12): p. 1199–1208.

4. Manworren, R., Mandatory continuing education for opioid prescribers. *Pain Medicine*, 2013. Nov 8 [epub ahead of print].

5. Johnson, M., B. Collett, and J.M. Castro-Lopes, The challenges of pain management in primary care: A pan-European survey. *J Pain Res*, 2013. **6**: p. 393–401.

6. Schubert, I., Ihle, P., Sabatowski, R., Increase in opiate prescription in Germany between 2000 and 2010. *Deutsches Arzteblatt International*, 2013. **110**(4): p. 45–51.

7. Kissin, I., Long-term opioid treatment of chronic nonmalignant pain: Unproven efficacy and neglected safety? *J Pain Res*, 2013. **6**: p. 513–29.

8. Chaparro, L.E., et al., Opioids compared to placebo or other treatments for chronic low-back pain. *Cochrane Database Syst Rev*, 2013. **8**: p. CD004959.

9. Kalso, E., et al., Opioids in chronic non-cancer pain: Systematic review of efficacy and safety. *Pain*, 2004. **112**(3): p. 372–80.

10. Anastassopoulos, K.P., et al., Economic study on the impact of side effects in patients taking oxycodone controlled-release for noncancer pain. *J Manag Care Pharm*, 2012. **18**(8): p. 615–26.

11. Darnall, B.D., B.R. Stacey, and R. Chou, Medical and psychological risks and consequences of long term opioid use in women (comprehensive review). *Pain Medicine*, 2012(Sept): p. 1181–1211.

12. Darnall, B.D., and B.R. Stacey, Sex differences examined in long-term opioid use: Cautionary notes for prescribing in women. *Archives of Internal Medicine*, 2012. **172**(5: 431–2).

13. Furlan, A., et al., A comparison between enriched and nonenriched enrollment randomized withdrawal trials of opioids for chronic noncancer pain. *Pain Research & Management*, 2011. **16**(5): p. 337–51.

14. Von Korff, M. Opioids for chronic pain: The status quo is not an option. *Northwest Regional Primary Care Association*. www.nwrpca.org/health-center-news/246-opioids-for-chronic-pain-the-status-quo-is-not-an-option.html [accessed 2012 December].

15. McWilliams, L.A., B.J. Cox, and M.W. Enns, Mood and anxiety disorders associated with chronic pain: An examination in a nationally representative sample. *Pain*, 2003. **106**(1–2): p. 127–33.

16. Younger, J.W., et al., Prescription opioid analgesics rapidly change the human brain. *Pain*, 2011. **152**(8): p. 1803–10.

17. Fanoe, S., et al., Oxycodone is associated with dose-dependent QTc prolongation in patients and low-affinity inhibiting of hERG activity in vitro. *Br J Clin Pharmacol*, 2009. **67**(2): p. 172–9.

18. Benton, R.E., et al., Greater quinidine-induced QTc interval prolongation in women. *Clin Pharmacol Ther*, 2000. **67**(4): p. 413–8.

19. Tompkins, D.A., et al., Concurrent validation of the Clinical Opiate Withdrawal Scale (COWS) and single-item indices against the Clinical Institute Narcotic Assessment (CINA) opioid withdrawal instrument. *Drug & Alcohol Dependence*, 2009. **105**(1–2): p. 154–9.

20. Wikipedia, Opioid dependence [accessed 2012 October].

21. Jensen, M.K., A.B. Thomsen, and J. Hojsted, 10-year follow-up of chronic non-malignant pain patients: Opioid use, health related quality of life and health care utilization. *Eur J Pain*, 2006. **10**(5): p. 423–33.

22. Breckenridge, J., and J.D. Clark, Patient characteristics associated with opioid versus nonsteroidal anti-inflammatory drug management of chronic low back pain. *J Pain*, 2003. **4**(6): p. 344–50.

23. Ciccone, D.S., et al., Psychological correlates of opioid use in patients with chronic nonmalignant pain: A preliminary test of the downhill spiral hypothesis. *J Pain Symptom Manage*, 2000. **20**(3): p. 180–92.

24. Braden, J.B., et al., Trends in long-term opioid therapy for noncancer pain among persons with a history of depression. *Gen Hosp Psychiatry*, 2009. **31**(6): p. 564–70.

25. Le Merrer, J., et al., Reward processing by the opioid system in the brain. *Physiol Rev*, 2009. **89**(4): p. 1379–412.

26. Baker, K., M. Foti, L. Jastrazab, E. Stringer, S. Mackey, and J. Younger, Immediate and lasting improvements in depression following rapid opioid detoxification. *Journal of Pain*, 2013. **14**(4): p. S78.

27. Franklin, G.M., et al., Opioid use for chronic low back pain: A prospective, population-based study among injured workers in Washington state, 2002–2005. Clinical *Journal of Pain*, 2009. **25**(9): p. 743–51.

28. Luomajoki, H., et al., Improvement in low back movement control, decreased pain and disability, resulting from specific exercise intervention. *Sports Med Arthrosc Rehabil Ther Technol*, 2010. **2**: p. 11.

29. Jensen, I.B., et al., A randomized controlled component analysis of a behavioral medicine rehabilitation program for chronic spinal pain: Are the effects dependent on gender? *Pain*, 2001. **91**(1–2): p. 65–78.

30. McCracken, L.M., and D.C. Turk, Behavioral and cognitive-behavioral treatment for chronic pain: Outcome, predictors of outcome, and treatment process. *Spine (Phila Pa 1976)*, 2002. **27**(22): p. 2564–73.

31. Hawkes, N.D., et al., Naloxone treatment for irritable bowel syndrome— A randomized controlled trial with an oral formulation. *Alimentary Pharmacology & Therapeutics*, 2002. **16**(9): p. 1649–54.

32. Crofford, L.J., Adverse effects of chronic opioid therapy for chronic musculoskeletal pain. *Nat Rev Rheumatol*, 2010. **6**(4): p. 191–7.

33. Saper, J.R., and A.E. Lake, 3rd, Continuous opioid therapy (COT) is rarely advisable for refractory chronic daily headache: Limited efficacy, risks, and proposed guidelines. *Headache*, 2008. **48**(6): p. 838–49.

34. Abs, R., et al., Endocrine consequences of long-term intrathecal administration of opioids. *J Clin Endocrinol Metab*, 2000. **85**(6): p. 2215–22.

35. Bennett, R.M., et al., Impact of fibromyalgia pain on health-related quality of life before and after treatment with tramadol/acetaminophen. *Arthritis & Rheumatism*, 2005. **53**(4): p. 519–27.

36. Holman, A.J., and R.R. Myers, A randomized, double-blind, placebo-controlled trial of pramipexole, a dopamine agonist, in patients with fibromyalgia receiving concomitant medications. *Arthritis & Rheumatism*, 2005. **52**(8): p. 2495–505.

37. Ngian, G.-S., E.K. Guymer, and G.O. Littlejohn, The use of opioids in fibromyalgia. *International Journal of Rheumatic Diseases*, 2010. **14**(1): p. 6–11.

38. Painter, J.T., and L.J. Crofford, Chronic opioid use in fibromyalgia syndrome: A clinical review. *J Clin Rheumatol*, 2013. **19**(2): p. 72–7.

39. Buckley, D.I., et al., Chronic opioid therapy and preventive services in rural primary care: An Oregon rural practice-based research network study. *Ann Fam Med*, 2010. **8**(3): p. 237–44.

40. Dimsdale, J.E., et al., The effect of opioids on sleep architecture. *J Clin Sleep Med*, 2007. **3**(1): p. 33–6.

41. Alattar, M.A., and S.M. Scharf, Opioid-associated central sleep apnea: A case series. *Sleep & Breathing*, 2009. **13**(2): p. 201–6.

42. Guilleminault, C., et al., Obstructive sleep apnea and chronic opioid use. *Lung,* 2010. **188**(6): p. 459–68.

43. Walker, J.M., et al., Chronic opioid use is a risk factor for the development of central sleep apnea and ataxic breathing.. *Journal of Clinical Sleep Medicine,* 2007. **3**(5): p. 455–61. [Erratum appears in J Clin Sleep Med. 2007 Oct 15;3(6):table of contents]

44. Webster, L.R., et al., Sleep-disordered breathing and chronic opioid therapy. *Pain Medicine,* 2008. **9**(4): p. 425–32.

45. Al Lawati, N.M., S.R. Patel, and N.T. Ayas, Epidemiology, risk factors, and consequences of obstructive sleep apnea and short sleep duration. *Progress in Cardiovascular Diseases,* 2009. **51**(4): p. 285–93.

46. Ramar, K., Reversal of sleep-disordered breathing with opioid withdrawal. *Pain Practice,* 2009. **9**(5): p. 394–8.

47. Davis, M.J., M. Livingston, and S.M. Scharf, Reversal of central sleep apnea following discontinuation of opioids. *J Clin Sleep Med,* 2012. **8**(5): p. 579–80.

48. Ackerman, W.E., 3rd, and M. Ahmad, Effect of cigarette smoking on serum hydrocodone levels in chronic pain patients. *J Ark Med Soc,* 2007. **104**(1): p. 19–21.

49. Ekholm, O., et al., Alcohol and smoking behavior in chronic pain patients: The role of opioids. *Eur J Pain,* 2008.

50. Hooten, W.M., et al., The effects of depression and smoking on pain severity and opioid use in patients with chronic pain. *Pain,* 2011. **152**(1): p. 223–9.

51. Hooten, W.M., et al., Effects of smoking status on immediate treatment outcomes of multidisciplinary pain rehabilitation. *Pain Med,* 2009. **10**(2): p. 347–55.

52. Krebs, E.E., et al., Predictors of long-term opioid use among patients with painful lumbar spine conditions. *J Pain,* 2010. **11**(1): p. 44–52.

53. Stover, B.D., et al., Factors associated with early opioid prescription among workers with low back injuries. *J Pain,* 2006. **7**(10): p. 718–25.

54. Weingarten, T.N., V.R. Podduturu, W.M. Hooten, J.M. Thompson, C.A. Luedtke, and T.H. Oh, Impact of tobacco use in patients presenting to a multidisciplinary outpatient treatment program for fibromyalgia. *Clin J Pain,* 2009. **25**(1): p. 39–43.

55. Gupta, S., and R. Atcheson, Opioid and chronic non-cancer pain. *J Anaesthesiol Clin Pharmacol,* 2013. **29**(1): p. 6–12.

56. Dunn, K.M., et al., Opioid prescriptions for chronic pain and overdose: A cohort study. *Ann Intern Med,* 2010. **152**(2): p. 85–92.

57. Angst, M.S., and J.D. Clark, Opioid-induced hyperalgesia: A qualitative systematic review. *Anesthesiology,* 2006. **104**(3): p. 570–87.

58. Bannister, K., and A.H. Dickenson, Opioid hyperalgesia. *Current Opinion in Supportive & Palliative Care*, 2010. **4**(1): p. 1–5.

59. Chu, L.F., M.S. Angst, and D. Clark, Opioid-induced hyperalgesia in humans: Molecular mechanisms and clinical considerations. *Clinical Journal of Pain*, 2008. **24**(6): p. 479–96.

60. Chu, L.F., D.J. Clark, and M.S. Angst, Opioid tolerance and hyperalgesia in chronic pain patients after one month of oral morphine therapy: A preliminary prospective study. *Journal of Pain*, 2006. **7**(1): p. 43–8.

61. Fishbain, D.A., et al., Do opioids induce hyperalgesia in humans? An evidence-based structured review. *Pain Med*, 2009. **10**(5): p. 829–39.

62. Baron, M.J., and P.W. McDonald, Significant pain reduction in chronic pain patients after detoxification from high-dose opioids. *Journal of Opioid Management*, 2006. **2**(5): p. 277–82.

63. Daniell, H.W., Hypogonadism in men consuming sustained-action oral opioids. *J Pain*, 2002. **3**(5): p. 377–84.

64. Brennan, M.J., The effect of opioid therapy on endocrine function. *Am J Med*, 2013. **126**(3 Suppl 1): p. S12–8.

65. Handal, M., et al., Use of prescribed opioid analgesics and co-medication with benzodiazepines in women before, during, and after pregnancy: A population-based cohort study. *Eur J Clin Pharmacol*, 2011. **67**(9): p. 953–60.

66. Madadi, P., et al., Genetic transmission of cytochrome P450 2D6 (CYP2D6) ultrarapid metabolism: Implications for breastfeeding women taking codeine. *Curr Drug Saf*, 2011. **6**(1): p. 36–9.

67. Madadi, P., et al., Safety of codeine during breastfeeding: Fatal morphine poisoning in the breastfed neonate of a mother prescribed codeine. *Can Fam Physician*, 2007. **53**(1): p. 33–5.

68. Madadi, P., et al., Guidelines for maternal codeine use during breastfeeding. *Can Fam Physician*, 2009. **55**(11): p. 1077–8.

69. Madadi, P., et al., Pharmacogenetics of neonatal opioid toxicity following maternal use of codeine during breastfeeding: A case-control study. *Clin Pharmacol Ther*, 2009. **85**(1): p. 31–5.

70. Madadi, P., et al., Establishing causality of CNS depression in breastfed infants following maternal codeine use. *Paediatr Drugs*, 2008. **10**(6): p. 399–404.

71. Daniell, H.W., Opioid endocrinopathy in women consuming prescribed sustained-action opioids for control of nonmalignant pain. *J Pain*, 2008. **9**(1): p. 28–36.

72. Rhodin, A., M. Stridsberg, and T. Gordh, Opioid endocrinopathy: A clinical problem in patients with chronic pain and long-term oral opioid treatment. *Clin J Pain*, 2010. **26**(5): p. 374–80.

73. Vuong, C., et al., The effects of opioids and opioid analogs on animal and human endocrine systems. *Endocr Rev*, 2010. **31**(1): p. 98–132.

74. Broussard, C.S., et al., Maternal treatment with opioid analgesics and risk for birth defects. *Am J Obstet Gynecol*, 2011. **204**(4): p. 314 e1–e11.

75. Boneva, R.S., et al., Mortality associated with congenital heart defects in the United States: Trends and racial disparities, 1979–1997. *Circulation*, 2001. **103**(19): p. 2376–81.

76. Saunders, K.W., et al., Relationship of opioid use and dosage levels to fractures in older chronic pain patients. *J Gen Intern Med*, 2010. **25**(4): p. 310–5.

77. Roth, S.H., et al., Around-the-clock, controlled-release oxycodone therapy for osteoarthritis-related pain: Placebo-controlled trial and long-term evaluation. *Arch Intern Med*, 2000. **160**(6): p. 853–60.

78. Miller, M., et al., Opioid analgesics and the risk of fractures in older adults with arthritis. *J Am Geriatr Soc*. **59**(3): p. 430–8.

79. Campbell, C.I., et al., Age and gender trends in long-term opioid analgesic use for noncancer pain. *Am J Public Health*, 2010. **100**(12): p. 2541–7.

80. Crisostomo, R.A., et al., Withdrawal of analgesic medication for chronic low-back pain patients: Improvement in outcomes of multidisciplinary rehabilitation regardless of surgical history. *Am J Phys Med Rehabil*, 2008. **87**(7): p. 527–36.

81. Murphy, J.L., M.E. Clark, and E. Banou, Opioid cessation and multidimensional outcomes after interdisciplinary chronic pain treatment. *Clin J Pain*, 2013. **29**(2): p. 109–17.

82. Bekhit, M.H., Opioid-induced hyperalgesia and tolerance. *American Journal of Therapeutics*, 2010. **17**(5): p. 498–510.

83. Lee, M., et al., A comprehensive review of opioid-induced hyperalgesia. *Pain Physician*, 2011. **14**(2): p. 145–61.

84. Chen, L., et al., Altered quantitative sensory testing outcome in subjects with opioid therapy. *Pain*, 2009. **143**(1–2): p. 65–70.

85. Colvin, L.A., and M.T. Fallon, Opioid-induced hyperalgesia: A clinical challenge. *British Journal of Anaesthesia*, 2010. **104**(2): p. 125–7.

86. Gardell, L.R., et al., Opioid receptor-mediated hyperalgesia and antinociceptive tolerance induced by sustained opiate delivery. *Neurosci Lett*, 2006. **396**(1): p. 44–9.

87. Holtman, J.R., Jr., and E.P. Wala, Characterization of morphine-induced hyperalgesia in male and female rats. *Pain*, 2005. **114**(1–2): p. 62–70.

88. Holtman, J.R., Jr., and E.P. Wala, Characterization of the antinociceptive effect of oxycodone in male and female rats. *Pharmacol Biochem Behav*, 2006. **83**(1): p. 100–8.

89. Ossipov, M.H., et al., Underlying mechanisms of pronociceptive consequences of prolonged morphine exposure. *Biopolymers,* 2005. **80**(2–3): p. 319–24.

90. Ballard, K.A., et al., Enhanced immune sensitivity to stress following chronic morphine exposure. *J Neuroimmune Pharmacol,* 2006. **1**(1): p. 106–15.

91. Hutchinson, M.R., et al., Exploring the neuroimmunopharmacology of opioids: An integrative review of mechanisms of central immune signaling and their implications for opioid analgesia. *Pharmacol Rev,* 2011. **63**(3): p. 772–810.

92. Sommer, C., and M. Kress, Recent findings on how proinflammatory cytokines cause pain: Peripheral mechanisms in inflammatory and neuropathic hyperalgesia. *Neurosci Lett,* 2004. **361**(1–3): p. 184–7.

93. Dina, O.A., P.G. Green, and J.D. Levine, Role of interleukin-6 in chronic muscle hyperalgesic priming. *Neuroscience,* 2008. **152**(2): p. 521–5.

94. De Jongh, R.F., et al., The role of interleukin-6 in nociception and pain. *Anesth Analg,* 2003. **96**(4): p. 1096–103, table of contents.

95. Bennett, R.M., et al., Tramadol and acetaminophen combination tablets in the treatment of fibromyalgia pain: A double-blind, randomized, placebo-controlled study. *American Journal of Medicine,* 2003. **114**(7): p. 537–45.

96. Pain. In *Merriam-Webster.com,* 2012.

97. Sullivan, M.D., et al., Regular use of prescribed opioids: Association with common psychiatric disorders. *Pain,* 2005. **119**(1–3): p. 95–103.

98. Sullivan, M.D., and J.C. Ballantyne, What are we treating with long-term opioid therapy? *Arch Intern Med,* 2012. **172**(5): p. 433–4.

99. Casey, P.P., A.M. Feyer, and I.D. Cameron, Identifying predictors of early non-recovery in a compensation setting: The whiplash outcome study. *Injury,* 2011. **42**(1): p. 25–32.

100. Sullivan, M.J., M.E. Lynch, and A.J. Clark, Dimensions of catastrophic thinking associated with pain experience and disability in patients with neuropathic pain conditions. *Pain,* 2005. **113**(3): p. 310–5.

101. Bhat, A.A., et al., The role of helplessness, outcome expectation for exercise and literacy in predicting disability and symptoms in older adults with arthritis. *Patient Educ Couns,* 2010. **81**(1): p. 73–8.

102. Nijs, J., et al., Exercise performance and chronic pain in chronic fatigue syndrome: The role of pain catastrophizing. *Pain Med,* 2008. **9**(8): p. 1164–72.

103. Crettaz, B., et al., Stress-induced allodynia—Evidence of increased pain sensitivity in healthy humans and patients with chronic pain after

experimentally induced psychosocial stress. *PLoS One,* 2013. **8**(8): p. e69460.

104. Burklund, L.J., N.I. Eisenberger, and M.D. Lieberman, The face of rejection: Rejection sensitivity moderates dorsal anterior cingulate activity to disapproving facial expressions. *Soc Neurosci,* 2007. **2**(3–4): p. 238–53.

105. Eisenberger, N.I., et al., An experimental study of shared sensitivity to physical pain and social rejection. *Pain,* 2006. **126**(1–3): p. 132–8.

106. Eisenberger, N.I., and M.D. Lieberman, Why rejection hurts: A common neural alarm system for physical and social pain. *Trends Cogn Sci,* 2004. **8**(7): p. 294–300.

107. Eisenberger, N.I., M.D. Lieberman, and K.D. Williams, Does rejection hurt?
An FMRI study of social exclusion. *Science,* 2003. **302**(5643): p. 290–2.

108. Eisenberger, N.I., The neural bases of social pain: Evidence for shared representations with physical pain. *Psychosom Med,* 2012. **74**(2): p. 126–35.

109. Eisenberger, N.I., The pain of social disconnection: Examining the shared neural underpinnings of physical and social pain. *Nat Rev Neurosci,* 2012. **13**(6): p. 421–34.

110. Steptoe, A., M. Hamer, and Y. Chida, The effects of acute psychological stress on circulating inflammatory factors in humans: A review and meta-analysis. *Brain Behav Immun,* 2007. **21**(7): p. 901–12.

111. Geiss, A., et al., Psychoneuroimmunological correlates of persisting sciatic pain in patients who underwent discectomy. *Neurosci Lett,* 1997. **237**(2–3): p. 65–8.

112. Koch, A., et al., Nitric oxide and pro-inflammatory cytokines correlate with pain intensity in chronic pain patients. *Inflamm Res,* 2007. **56**(1): p. 32–7.

113. Ludwig, J., et al., Cytokine expression in serum and cerebrospinal fluid in non-inflammatory polyneuropathies. *J Neurol Neurosurg Psychiatry,* 2008. 79:1269-1274.

114. Lutz, A., et al., Long-term meditators self-induce high-amplitude gamma synchrony during mental practice. *Proc Natl Acad Sci USA,* 2004. **101**(46): p. 16369–73.

115. Varela, F., et al., The brainweb: Phase synchronization and large-scale integration. *Nat Rev Neurosci,* 2001. **2**(4): p. 229–39.

116. Zaehle, T., and C.S. Herrmann, Neural synchrony and white matter variations in the human brain—Relation between evoked gamma frequency and corpus callosum morphology. *Int J Psychophysiol,* 2011. **79**: p. 49–54.

117. Jensen, O., R. Hari, and K. Kaila, Visually evoked gamma responses in the human brain are enhanced during voluntary hyperventilation. *Neuroimage*, 2002. **15**(3): p. 575–86.

118. Oster, G., Auditory beats in the brain. *Scientific American*, 1973. **229**(4): p. 94–102.

119. Kliempt, P., et al., Hemispheric-synchronisation during anaesthesia: A double-blind randomised trial using audiotapes for intra-operative nociception control. *Anaesthesia*, 1999. **54**(8): p. 769–73.

120. Lewis, A.K., I.P. Osborn, and R. Roth, The effect of hemispheric synchronization on intraoperative analgesia. *Anesth Analg*, 2004. **98**(2): p. 533–6, table of contents.

121. Lyle, K.B., and J.M. Martin, Bilateral saccades increase intrahemispheric processing but not interhemispheric interaction: Implications for saccade-induced retrieval enhancement. *Brain Cogn.* **73**(2): p. 128–34.

122. Bingel, U., et al., The effect of treatment expectation on drug efficacy: Imaging the analgesic benefit of the opioid remifentanil. *Sci Transl Med*, 2011. **3**(70): p. 70ra14.

123. Treede, R.D., et al., Cortical representation of pain: Functional characterization of nociceptive areas near the lateral sulcus. *Pain*, 2000. **87**(2): p. 113–9.

124. Melzack, R., From the gate to the neuromatrix. *Pain*, 1999. **Suppl 6**: p. S121–6.

125. Ploner, M., et al., Flexible cerebral connectivity patterns subserve contextual modulations of pain. *Cereb Cortex*, 2010. 21(3): p. 719–26.

126. Ploner, M., et al., Prestimulus functional connectivity determines pain perception in humans. *Proc Natl Acad Sci USA*, 2010. **107**(1): p. 355–60.

127. Wager, T.D., et al., Placebo-induced changes in FMRI in the anticipation and experience of pain. *Science*, 2004. **303**(5661): p. 1162–7.

128. Wager, T.D., et al., Predicting individual differences in placebo analgesia: Contributions of brain activity during anticipation and pain experience. *J Neurosci*, 2011. **31**(2): p. 439–52.

129. Sullivan, M.J.L., The pain catastrophizing scale: Development and validation. *Psychological Assessment*, 1995. **7**(4): p. 524–32.

130. Severeijns, R., et al., Pain catastrophizing predicts pain intensity, disability, and psychological distress independent of the level of physical impairment. *Clin J Pain*, 2001. **17**(2): p. 165–72.

131. George, S.Z., and A.T. Hirsh, Psychologic influence on experimental pain sensitivity and clinical pain intensity for patients with shoulder pain. *J Pain*, 2009. 10(3):p. 293–99.

132. Khan, R.S., et al., Catastrophizing: A predictive factor for postoperative pain. *Am J Surg*, 2011. **201**(1): p. 122–31.

133. Riddle, D.L., et al., Preoperative pain catastrophizing predicts pain outcome after knee arthroplasty. *Clin Orthop Relat Res*, 2010. **468**(3): p. 798–806.

134. Cook, A.J., P.A. Brawer, and K.E. Vowles, The fear-avoidance model of chronic pain: Validation and age analysis using structural equation modeling. *Pain*, 2006. **121**(3): p. 195–206.

135. Spinhoven, P., et al., Catastrophizing and internal pain control as mediators of outcome in the multidisciplinary treatment of chronic low back pain. *Eur J Pain*, 2004. **8**(3): p. 211–9.

136. Jensen, M.P., J.A. Turner, and J.M. Romano, Changes in beliefs, catastrophizing, and coping are associated with improvement in multidisciplinary pain treatment. *J Consult Clin Psychol*, 2001. **69**(4): p. 655–62.

137. Geisser, M.E., et al., Perception of noxious and innocuous heat stimulation among healthy women and women with fibromyalgia: Association with mood, somatic focus, and catastrophizing. *Pain*, 2003. **102**(3): p. 243–50.

138. Picavet, H.S., J.W. Vlaeyen, and J.S. Schouten, Pain catastrophizing and kinesiophobia: Predictors of chronic low back pain. *Am J Epidemiol*, 2002. **156**(11): p. 1028–34.

139. Burton, A.K., et al., Psychosocial predictors of outcome in acute and subchronic low back trouble. *Spine*, 1995. **20**(6): p. 722–8.

140. Ohara, S., et al., Analysis of synchrony demonstrates that the presence of "pain networks" prior to a noxious stimulus can enable the perception of pain in response to that stimulus. *Exp Brain Res*, 2008. **185**(2): p. 353–8.

141. Ohara, S., et al., Analysis of synchrony demonstrates 'pain networks' defined by rapidly switching, task-specific, functional connectivity between pain-related cortical structures. *Pain*, 2006. **123**(3): p. 244–53.

142. Seminowicz, D.A., and K.D. Davis, Cortical responses to pain in healthy individuals depends on pain catastrophizing. *Pain*, 2006. **120**(3): p. 297–306.

143. Gracely, R.H., et al., Pain catastrophizing and neural responses to pain among persons with fibromyalgia. *Brain*, 2004. **127**(Pt 4): p. 835–43.

144. Apkarian, A.V., Cortical pathophysiology of chronic pain. *Novartis Found Symp*, 2004. **261**: p. 239–45; discussion 245–61.

145. Apkarian, A.V., Pain perception in relation to emotional learning. *Curr Opin Neurobiol*, 2008. **18**(4): p. 464–8.

146. Apkarian, A.V., et al., Chronic pain patients are impaired on an emotional decision-making task. *Pain*, 2004. **108**(1–2): p. 129–36.

147. Apkarian, A.V., et al., Chronic back pain is associated with decreased prefrontal and thalamic gray matter density. *J Neurosci,* 2004. **24**(46): p. 10410–5.

148. Baliki, M.N., et al., Chronic pain and the emotional brain: Specific brain activity associated with spontaneous fluctuations of intensity of chronic back pain. *J Neurosci,* 2006. **26**(47): p. 12165–73.

149. Edwards, R.R., et al., Association of catastrophizing with interleukin-6 responses to acute pain. *Pain,* 2008. **140**(1): p. 135–44.

150. Darnall, B.D., M. Aickin, and H. Zwickey, Pilot study of inflammatory responses following a negative imaginal focus in persons with chronic pain: Analysis by sex/gender. *Gender Medicine,* 2010. **7**(3): p. 247–60.

151. Macedo, L.G., G.P. Bostick, and C.G. Maher, Exercise for prevention of recurrences of nonspecific low back pain. *Phys Ther,* 2013. 93(12):p. 1-6.

152. Olivier, N., et al., An exercise therapy program can increase oxygenation and blood volume of the erector spinae muscle during exercise in chronic low back pain patients. *Arch Phys Med Rehabil,* 2013. **94**(3): p. 536–42.

153. Thompson, J.M., Exercise in muscle pain disorders. *Phys Med Rehabil,* 2012. **4**(11): p. 889–93.

154. Ochsner, K.N., et al., Neural correlates of individual differences in pain-related fear and anxiety. *Pain,* 2006. **120**(1–2): p. 69–77.

155. Meier, B., and A. Goodnough, Administration wants tighter painkiller rules, in *New York Times,* 2011: New York (April 19, 2011)

156. Gabay, C., Interleukin-6 and chronic inflammation. *Arthritis Res Ther,* 2006. **8 Suppl 2**: p. S3.

157. Bhasin, M.K., et al., Relaxation response induces temporal transcriptome changes in energy metabolism, insulin secretion and inflammatory pathways. *PloS One,* 2013. May 1;8(5):e62817.

Index

Note: Page numbers followed by "f" and "t" indicate figures and tables, respectively.

IASP. *See* International Association for the Study of Pain (IASP)
Iatrogenic effects, 71n
IBD. *See* Irritable bowel disorder (IBD)
IBS. *See* Irritable bowel disorder (IBD)
Infants, breast-feeding, 46–47
Infertility, 47
Inflammation, 45, 48, 65–66, 65n, 100, 129
Inflammatory factors, 98, 100, 129
Inpatient detoxification programs, 172, 175–76
Insomnia. *See* Sleep problems
International Association for the Study of Pain (IASP), 80
Irritability, 43, 45, 52
Irritable bowel disorder (IBD), 23, 30
Irritable bowel syndrome (IBS). *See* Irritable bowel disorder (IBD)
Isoptin (verapamil), 28*t*

Jaqui, 8–11
Joan, 58–59, 66–68, 67–70, 71
Joann, 135
Jobs, 29
Joe, 57–58
Joint Commission, 15, 15n

Kadian, 200
Ketoconazole (Nizoral), 28*t*
Kirkegaard, Soren, *, 153
Klonopin (clonazepam), 28*t*, 42*t*

Ledger, Heath, 199, 199n
Lethargy, 45
Libido, low, 45, 48
Long QT syndrome, 22–23
Lorazepam (Ativan), 28*t*, 42*t*, 43, 56
Luis, 193–96, 194–95*t*
Lunesta, 43
Luteinizing hormone, 47–48, 47n

Matthew, 134–35, 140
Mayo Clinic, 38
McDonald, P.W., 67n
Medical education, 6–7, 197

Medical journals, publications in, 14–15
Medication, reducing, 169–71, 173, 186*t*
Medication trials, 51
Meditation, 106, 107–8
Meier, Barry, 199n
Memory problems, 66–67
Men, 20
 older, 49–50
 risks for, 45–46, 49–50
Menstrual cycle, loss of, 47
Meredith, 142–44
Methadone, 23, 200
 risks of, 32–33, 37
Migraines, 30–31, 142–43
 prevention of, 31–32
 treatment of, 31–32
Mind, the. *See also* Brain, the; Mind–body communication; Psychology, power of, 97
Mind–body communication, 83–84, 97, 100, 132, 145–46
Mind–body skills, 172
MiraLAX, 23
Mood problems, 17, 17*f*, 43, 45, 48. *See also* Irritability
Morphine, extended-release, 76
MS Contin, 200
Multidisciplinary pain treatment, 62
Murphy, Brittany, 199, 199n
Musculoskeletal pain, 30

Negative thoughts, 97, 121–29, 146–47, 149. *See also* Catastrophizing
Neonatal risks of opioids, 48–49
Nervous system, calming, 97–118
Neuropathic pain, 57
Neuroplasticity, 107
Neurostimulation, 36
New prescriptions, 43–44
Nizoral (ketoconazole), 28*t*
Nonsteroidal anti-inflammatory drugs (NSAIDs), 14, 46
Nortriptyline (Pamelor), 28*t*
NSAIDs. *See* Nonsteroidal anti-inflammatory drugs (NSAIDs)
Nucynta ER, 200

About the Author

Beth Darnall, PhD, is clinical professor at Stanford University in the Department of Anesthesiology, Perioperative and Pain Medicine, and, by courtesy, Psychiatry and Behavioral Sciences. She is principal investigator for nationally funded pain and opioid reduction research projects that include psychological treatment approaches. She investigates targeted pain psychology treatments she has developed to reduce post-surgical pain and opioid use and community-based, patient-centered opioid tapering. She speaks nationally and internationally on pain and opioid reduction. She also authored *The Opioid-Free Pain Relief Kit* ©2016 (Bull Publishing) and *Psychological Treatment for Patients with Chronic Pain* ©2018 (American Psychological Association Press). She spoke on the psychology of pain relief at the 2018 World Economic Forum in Davos, Switzerland, and has been featured in major media outlets, including *O Magazine, Forbes, Scientific American, The Washington Post, BBC Radio, Nature,* and *TIME Magazine.*

Website: bethdarnall.com
Twitter: @bethdarnall

1